# Obstructive Sleep Apnea

*Editor*

MARK A. D'AGOSTINO

# OTOLARYNGOLOGIC CLINICS OF NORTH AMERICA

www.oto.theclinics.com

December 2016 • Volume 49 • Number 6

**ELSEVIER**

1600 John F. Kennedy Boulevard • Suite 1800 • Philadelphia, Pennsylvania, 19103-2899

http://www.oto.theclinics.com

OTOLARYNGOLOGIC CLINICS OF NORTH AMERICA Volume 49, Number 6
December 2016 ISSN 0030-6665, ISBN-13: 978-0-323-47746-8

Editor: Jessica McCool
Developmental Editor: Alison Swety

*Otolaryngologic Clinics of North America* (ISSN 0030-6665) is published bimonthly by Elsevier, Inc., 360 Park Avenue South, New York, NY 10010-1710. Months of issue are February, April, June, August, October, and December. Business and Editorial Offices: 1600 John F. Kennedy Blvd., Suite 1800, Philadelphia, PA 19103-2899. Customer Service Office: 6277 Sea Harbor Drive, Orlando, FL 32887-4800. Periodicals postage paid at New York, NY and additional mailing offices. Subscription prices are $370.00 per year (US individuals), $765.00 per year (US institutions), $100.00 per year (US student/resident), $485.00 per year (Canadian individuals), $969.00 per year (Canadian institutions), $540.00 per year (international individuals), $969.00 per year (international institutions), $270.00 per year (international & Canadian student/resident). Foreign air speed delivery is included in all *Clinics'* subscription prices. All prices are subject to change without notice. **POSTMASTER:** Send address changes to *Otolaryngologic Clinics of North America*, Elsevier Health Sciences Division, Subscription Customer Service, 3251 Riverport Lane, Maryland Heights, MO 63043. **Telephone: 1-800-654-2452 (U.S. and Canada); 314-447-8871 (outside U.S. and Canada). Fax: 314-447-8029. E-mail: journalscustomerservice-usa@elsevier.com (for print support); journalsonlinesupport-usa@elsevier.com (for online support).**

*Reprints.* For copies of 100 or more of articles in this publication, please contact the Commercial Reprints Department, Elsevier Inc., 360 Park Avenue South, New York, NY 10010-1710. Tel.: 212-633-3874; Fax: 212-633-3820; E-mail: reprints@elsevier.com.

*Otolaryngologic Clinics of North America* is also published in Spanish by McGraw-Hill Interamericana Editores S.A., P.O. Box 5-237, 06500 Mexico D.F., Mexico.

*Otolaryngologic Clinics of North America* is covered in *MEDLINE/PubMed (Index Medicus), Current Contents/Clinical Medicine, Excerpta Medica, BIOSIS, Science Citation Index,* and *ISI/BIOMED.*

## PROGRAM OBJECTIVE
The goal of the *Otolaryngologic Clinics of North America* is to provide information on the latest trends in patient management, the newest advances; and provide a sound basis for choosing treatment options in the field of otolaryngology.

## LEARNING OBJECTIVES
Upon completion of this activity, participants will be able to:
1. Review obstructive sleep apnea in children and adults.
2. Discuss surgical options in the treatment of obstructive sleep apnea.
3. Recognize therapies, procedures, and appliances used for treatment of obstructive sleep apnea.

## ACCREDITATION
The Elsevier Office of Continuing Medical Education (EOCME) is accredited by the Accreditation Council for Continuing Medical Education (ACCME) to provide continuing medical education for physicians.

The EOCME designates this enduring material for a maximum of 15 *AMA PRA Category 1 Credit*(s)™. Physicians should claim only the credit commensurate with the extent of their participation in the activity.

All other health care professionals requesting continuing education credit for this enduring material will be issued a certificate of participation.

## DISCLOSURE OF CONFLICTS OF INTEREST
The EOCME assesses conflict of interest with its instructors, faculty, planners, and other individuals who are in a position to control the content of CME activities. All relevant conflicts of interest that are identified are thoroughly vetted by EOCME for fair balance, scientific objectivity, and patient care recommendations. EOCME is committed to providing its learners with CME activities that promote improvements or quality in healthcare and not a specific proprietary business or a commercial interest.

**The planning committee, staff, authors and editors listed below have identified no financial relationships or relationships to products or devices they or their spouse/life partner have with commercial interest related to the content of this CME activity:**
Moh'd Al-Halawani, MD; José E. Barrera, MD, FACS; Adrianne Brigido; Natamon Charakorn, MD; Mark A. D'Agostino, MD, FACS; Anthony Dioguardi, DMD; Jeffrey Dorrity, MD; Zarmina Ehsan, MD; Anjali Fortna; Katherine Koral Green, MD, MS; David Hamlar, MD, DDS; Stacey L. Ishman, MD, MPH; Eric J. Kezirian, MD, MPH; Jessica McCool; Premkumar Nandhakumar; Boris Paskhover, MD; Lee Shangold, MD, FACS; Megan Suermann; Alison Swety; Pnina Weiss, MD; Nicholas Wirtz, MD; Kathleen Yaremchuk, MD, MSA.

**The planning committee, staff, authors and editors listed below have identified financial relationships or relationships to products or devices they or their spouse/life partner have with commercial interest related to the content of this CME activity:**
**Oleg Froymovich, MD** is a consultant/advisor for Medtronic.
**Meir Kryger, MD, FRCPC** has research support from Koninklijke Philips N.V. and Resmed, and is a consultant/advisor for Inspire Pharmaceuticals, Inc, now part of Merck & Co., Inc.
**Samuel A. Mickelson, MD, FACS, FABSM** is a consultant/advisor for, and has stock ownership in, Zelegent, Inc. and Siesta Medical, Inc, and has research support from Inspire Pharmaceuticals, Inc, now part of Merck & Co., Inc., and ImThera Medical.
**B. Tucker Woodson, MD** is a consultant/advisor for Inspire Pharmaceuticals, Inc, now part of Merck & Co., Inc., and Medtronic, has stock ownership in Zelegent, Inc. and Siesta Medical, Inc, has research support from Inspire Pharmaceuticals, Inc, now part of Merck & Co., Inc., and receives royalties/patents from Medtronic. His spouse/partner is a consultant/advisor for Zelegent, Inc.; Lingualflex, Inc, and Cryosa.

## UNAPPROVED/OFF-LABEL USE DISCLOSURE
The EOCME requires CME faculty to disclose to the participants:
1. When products or procedures being discussed are off-label, unlabelled, experimental, and/or investigational (not US Food and Drug Administration [FDA] approved); and
2. Any limitations on the information presented, such as data that are preliminary or that represent ongoing research, interim analyses, and/or unsupported opinions. Faculty may discuss information about pharmaceutical agents that is outside of FDA-approved labelling. This information is intended solely for CME and is not intended to promote off-label use of these medications. If you have any questions, contact the medical affairs department of the manufacturer for the most recent prescribing information.

## TO ENROLL

To enroll in the *Otolaryngologic Clinics of North America* Continuing Medical Education program, call customer service at 1-800-654-2452 or sign up online at http://www.theclinics.com/home/cme. The CME program is available to subscribers for an additional annual fee of USD 260.

## METHOD OF PARTICIPATION

In order to claim credit, participants must complete the following:

1. Complete enrolment as indicated above.
2. Read the activity.
3. Complete the CME Test and Evaluation. Participants must achieve a score of 70% on the test. All CME Tests and Evaluations must be completed online.

## CME INQUIRIES/SPECIAL NEEDS

For all CME inquiries or special needs, please contact elsevierCME@elsevier.com.

# Contributors

## EDITOR

**MARK A. D'AGOSTINO, MD, FACS**
Partner/Owner, Southern New England Ear, Nose, Throat and Facial Plastic Surgery Group, New Haven, Connecticut; Assistant Professor of Surgery, Frank H. Netter MD School of Medicine, Quinnipiac University, North Haven, Connecticut; Clinical Instructor, Section of Otolaryngology, Yale School of Medicine, Yale University, New Haven, Connecticut; Assistant Professor of Surgery, F. Edward Hebert School of Medicine, Uniformed Services University of the Health Sciences, Bethesda, Maryland; Chief of Otolaryngology Section, Middlesex Hospital, Middletown, Connecticut

## AUTHORS

**MOH'D AL-HALAWANI, MD**
Sleep Medicine Fellowship Program, Section of Pulmonary, Critical Care and Sleep Medicine, Yale School of Medicine, Yale University, New Haven, Connecticut

**JOSÉ E. BARRERA, MD, FACS**
Associate Professor, Uniformed Services University of the Health Sciences, Bethesda, Maryland; Clinical Associate Professor, University of Texas Health Sciences Center; Medical Director, Texas Facial Plastic Surgery and ENT, San Antonio, Texas

**NATAMON CHARAKORN, MD**
Department of Otolaryngology – Head and Neck Surgery, Faculty of Medicine, King Chulalonkorn Memorial Hospital, Chulalongkorn University, Thai Red Cross Society, Bangkok, Thailand

**MARK A. D'AGOSTINO, MD, FACS**
Partner/Owner, Southern New England Ear, Nose, Throat and Facial Plastic Surgery Group, New Haven, Connecticut; Assistant Professor of Surgery, Frank H. Netter MD School of Medicine, Quinnipiac University, North Haven, Connecticut; Clinical Instructor, Section of Otolaryngology, Yale School of Medicine, Yale University, New Haven, Connecticut; Assistant Professor of Surgery, F. Edward Hebert School of Medicine, Uniformed Services University of the Health Sciences, Bethesda, Maryland; Chief of Otolaryngology Section, Middlesex Hospital, Middletown, Connecticut

**ANTHONY DIOGUARDI, DMD**
Diplomate of the American Board of Dental Sleep Medicine, Dental Director, Sleep Apnea and Snoring Dental Therapy of Connecticut; Instructor, Yale University Sleep Medicine Fellowship Program; Attending Yale New Haven Hospital, Department of Dentistry, New Haven, Connecticut

**JEFFREY DORRITY, MD**
Resident, Department of Otolaryngology, University of Minnesota, Minneapolis, Minnesota

**ZARMINA EHSAN, MD**
Sleep Fellow, Division of Pulmonary Medicine, Cincinnati Children's Hospital Medical Center, Cincinnati, Ohio

**OLEG FROYMOVICH, MD**
Staff, Department of Otolaryngology, Paparella Ear Head & Neck Institute, University of Minnesota, Minneapolis, Minnesota

**KATHERINE KORAL GREEN, MD, MS**
Assistant Professor, Director of Sleep Surgery, Department of Otolaryngology – Head and Neck Surgery, University of Colorado School of Medicine, Aurora, Colorado

**DAVID HAMLAR, MD, DDS**
Assistant Professor, Department of Otolaryngology, University of Minnesota, Minneapolis, Minnesota

**STACEY L. ISHMAN, MD, MPH**
Professor, Divisions of Pulmonary Medicine and Pediatric Otolaryngology – Head & Neck Surgery, Surgical Director, Upper Airway Center, Cincinnati Children's Hospital Medical Center; Department of Otolaryngology – Head and Neck Surgery, University of Cincinnati School of Medicine, Cincinnati, Ohio

**ERIC J. KEZIRIAN, MD, MPH**
USC Caruso Department of Otolaryngology – Head and Neck Surgery, Keck School of Medicine of USC, Los Angeles, California

**MEIR KRYGER, MD, FRCPC**
Professor, Pulmonary, Critical Care and Sleep Medicine, Yale School of Medicine, Yale University, New Haven, Connecticut

**SAMUEL A. MICKELSON, MD, FACS, FABSM**
Advanced Ear Nose & Throat Associates, The Atlanta Snoring & Sleep Disorders Institute, Atlanta, Georgia

**BORIS PASKHOVER, MD**
Section of Otolaryngology, Yale School of Medicine, Yale University, New Haven, Connecticut

**LEE SHANGOLD, MD, FACS**
ENT and Allergy Associates, Port Jefferson Station, New York

**PNINA WEISS, MD**
Associate Professor, Pediatric Respiratory Medicine and Medical Education, Yale School of Medicine, Yale University, New Haven, Connecticut

**NICHOLAS WIRTZ, MD**
Resident, Department of Otolaryngology, University of Minnesota, Minneapolis, Minnesota

**B. TUCKER WOODSON, MD**
Professor and Chief, Division of Sleep Medicine and Surgery, Department of Otolaryngology, Medical College Wisconsin, Milwaukee, Wisconsin

**KATHLEEN YAREMCHUK, MD, MSA**
Chair, Department of Otolaryngology – Head and Neck Surgery, Henry Ford Hospital; Clinical Professor, Department of Otolaryngology – Head and Neck Surgery, Wayne State University School of Medicine, Detroit, Michigan

# Contents

Obstructive sleep apnea (OSA) is a prevalent disease entity that has become commonplace over the past few decades. Its surge in diagnosis can be linked to a better understanding of the process with a concurrent increase in prevalence. The social, economic, and personal impacts are significant; there continues to be a need to improve our treatment modalities for OSA.

There is more information on a sleep study report than just the Apnea-Hypopnea Index or Respiratory Disturbance Index. This article explains how to evaluate any sleep study report to get the most information out of it. Maximum information allows the optimal treatment of patients with obstructive sleep apnea and some other sleep disorders.

Positive airway pressure (PAP) is considered first-line therapy for moderate to severe obstructive sleep apnea and may also be considered for mild obstructive sleep apnea, particularly if it is symptomatic or there are concomitant cardiovascular disorders. Continuous PAP is most commonly used. Other modes, such as bilevel airway pressure, autotitrating positive airway pressure, average volume assured pressure support, and adaptive support ventilation, play important roles in the management of sleep-related breathing disorders. This article outlines the indications, description, and comfort features of each mode. Despite the proven efficacy of PAP in treating obstructive sleep apnea syndrome and its sequelae, adherence to therapy is low. Close follow-up of patients for evaluation of adherence to and effectiveness of treatment is important.

Oral appliance therapy (OAT) has become an increasingly popular nonsurgical option for the treatment of obstructive sleep disorders. Recent research supports its efficacy and high levels of compliance for patients with obstructive sleep disorders. Common side effects of OAT include temporomandibular joint–related symptoms, bite changes, and tooth

areas of the upper airway. Because of the wide variety of physiologic and anatomic causes of this disorder it is important to tailor the treatment to offer the patient the best possible outcome. Genioglossus, hyoid, and tongue base procedures should be considered among theses treatment options.

Mark A. D'Agostino

The standard treatment for patients with obstructive sleep apnea syndrome is positive airway pressure (PAP) therapy. However, when PAP therapy fails, surgery may be an option to alleviate the obstruction. The base of tongue plays an important role in this obstruction, and addressing the tongue base surgically can be a challenge for the head and neck surgeon. Transoral robotic surgery (TORS) using the da Vinci Surgical System provides a safe and effective way to approach and manage the base of tongue and supraglottis. Advantages of TORS include wide-field high-definition 3-D visualization, precise instrumentation, and when compared with open procedures, less operative time, quicker recovery, no external scars, and comparable tissue resection.

Katherine Koral Green and B. Tucker Woodson

Traditional upper airway surgery directly modifies skeletal and soft tissue structures surrounding the airway to treat obstructive sleep apnea (OSA). Upper airway stimulation (UAS) attempts to treat upper airway obstruction and OSA by stimulating the hypoglossal nerve. The Inspire II implant has been approved for clinical UAS. Basic science data support that UAS prevents obstruction and improves airflow. Clinical results demonstrate that UAS improves respiratory sleep metrics and improves both objective and subjective self-reported sleep and quality-of-life outcomes. In a substantial number of individuals who meet inclusion criteria, UAS appears to be a viable, long-term, low-morbidity treatment of moderate-to-severe OSA.

José E. Barrera

Multilevel surgery has been established as the mainstay of treatment for the surgical management of obstructive sleep apnea (OSA). Combined with uvulopalatopharyngoplasty, tongue-base surgeries, including the genioglossus advancement (GA), sliding genioplasty, and hyoid myotomy and suspension, have been developed to target hypopharyngeal obstruction. Total airway surgery consisting of maxillomandibular advancement (MMA) with/without GA has shown significant success. Skeletal procedures for OSA with or without a palatal procedure is a proven technique for relieving airway obstruction during sleep. A case study demonstrating the utility of virtual surgical planning for MMA surgery is presented.

Screening for obstructive sleep apnea (OSA) with in-laboratory polysomnography is recommended for children with sleep disordered breathing.
Adenotonsillectomy is the first-line therapy for pediatric OSA, although
intranasal steroids and montelukast can be considered for those with
mild OSA and continuous positive airway pressure for those with moderate
to severe OSA awaiting surgery, poor surgical candidates or persistent
OSA. Bony or soft tissue upper airway surgery is reasonable for children
failing medical management or those with persistent OSA following adenotonsillectomy. Weight loss and oral appliance therapy are also useful. A
multi-modality approach to diagnosis and treatment is preferred.

# OTOLARYNGOLOGIC CLINICS
# OF NORTH AMERICA

# Preface

# Obstructive Sleep Apnea, Diagnosis, Management, and Treatment

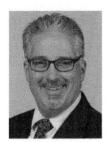

Mark A. D'Agostino MD, FACS
*Editor*

The incidence of sleep-disordered breathing, and specifically obstructive sleep apnea, has increased significantly over the last several decades. This increase parallels the increase in the rate of obesity seen in the United States over the same time frame. As Dr Paskhover points out in his introductory article, it has been estimated that the obesity rate in the United States has increased from 15% in 1990 to 36% in 2012.

The economic impact of untreated sleep apnea is staggering and is felt far and wide, not only on the amount of health care dollars spent on untreated apneic patients but also on its effect on the workforce in terms of decreased productivity, work days lost, and disability.

The health consequences of untreated apnea have become more and more apparent over the years. Untreated apnea can be associated with the development of cardiovascular disease (including hypertension, congestive heart failure, arrhythmias, and strokes), insulin resistance, cognitive impairment, and increased markers of inflammation.

I am pleased to present this issue of *Otolaryngologic Clinics of North America* dedicated to obstructive sleep apnea. I am honored to have assembled a group of national experts to discuss the diagnosis and treatment of patients with obstructive sleep apnea. In the following articles, we review the use of both in-lab and home sleep testing and the role of each in diagnosis, review the use of drug-induced sleep endoscopy to assess the collapsibility of the upper airway, and discuss the treatment options of positive airway pressure, oral appliances, and surgery. Obstructive sleep apnea in the pediatric population is also addressed.

The field of sleep surgery has grown rapidly over the last several years, from the classic uvulopalatoplasty initially described by Fujita to the numerous palatal procedures currently available to the otolaryngologist. Based on earlier studies by Scher and

Otolaryngol Clin N Am 49 (2016) xiii–xiv
http://dx.doi.org/10.1016/j.otc.2016.10.001
0030-6665/16/© 2016 Published by Elsevier Inc.

oto.theclinics.com

others, we have come to realize the importance of addressing the base of the tongue along with the palate when treating patients with apnea.

Numerous procedures to address the base of tongue have been developed and are addressed here. I am especially excited to present the latest advances in addressing the base of tongue, including transoral robotic partial glossectomy and hypoglossal nerve stimulation therapy.

Hypoglossal nerve stimulation therapy is a novel approach to obstructive sleep apnea and may revolutionize the way obstructive sleep apnea is treated.

There is no doubt that the field of sleep medicine, and specifically obstructive sleep apnea, will continue to grow, and the otolaryngologist will continue to play a pivotal role in diagnosing and treating these patients.

Mark A. D'Agostino, MD, FACS
Southern New England Ear, Nose
Throat and Facial Plastic Surgery Group
One Long Wharf Drive
Suite 302
New Haven, CT 06511, USA

Frank H. Netter MD School of Medicine
Quinnipiac University
North Haven, CT, USA

Yale School of Medicine
Yale University
New Haven, CT, USA

Middlesex Hospital
Middletown, CT, USA

E-mail address:
madago@comcast.net

# An Introduction to Obstructive Sleep Apnea

Boris Paskhover, MD*

## KEYWORDS

- OSA • Prevalence • Obesity • History

## KEY POINTS

- Obstructive sleep apnea (OSA) is a prevalent disease entity that has become commonplace over the past few decades.
- Its surge in diagnosis can be linked to a better understanding of the process with a concurrent increase in prevalence.
- The social, economic, and personal impacts are significant; there continues to be a need to improve our treatment modalities for OSA.

## PICKWICKIAN SYNDROME

With the ever-increasing media coverage of obstructive sleep apnea (OSA) and its disastrous long-term effects, it is hard to believe that this clinical entity has only been clearly identified and recognized for several decades. The first clear modern description of the syndrome was by Burwell[1] in 1956 in the publication entitled, "Extreme Obesity Associated with Alveolar Hypoventilation: A Pickwickian Syndrome." The report details a young obese boy whose appearance parallels Joe from Charles Dickens' The Posthumous Papers of the Pickwick Club (1837). Its unclear if this patient truly had OSA, and it took another decade before Gastaut and colleagues[2] in 1966 showed repeated apneas in obese patients and noted these nocturnal disturbances to possibly be linked to their daytime somnolence.

Interestingly it seems that multiple physicians, including Broadbent[3] and Caton[4], alluded to a several cases in the late nineteenth century with a general understanding that obstructive apneas occur while asleep.[5] Some physicians suspect that the early overdiagnosis of sleep disorders, such as narcolepsy, were actually cases of OSA.[5] Luckily, in the last few decades our understanding of the pathophysiology and treatment of OSA has progressed significantly with entire medical journals focused on it.

No disclosures or financial conflicts.
Section of Otolaryngology, Yale School of Medicine, 800 Howard Avenue, Fourth Floor, New Haven, CT 06519, USA
* 634 Rosemount Lane, West Haven, CT 06516.
E-mail address: Boris.Paskhover@yale.edu

Otolaryngol Clin N Am 49 (2016) 1303–1306
http://dx.doi.org/10.1016/j.otc.2016.07.007     oto.theclinics.com

## INCREASING PREVALENCE

This increased focus on OSA is well justified with the noted increase in its prevalence. Franklin and Linderberg[6] showed in their review of the epidemiology of sleep apnea that the prevalence of the diagnosed entity with polysmonograms in epidemiologic studies to have increased significantly over the past 3 decades. An epidemiologic study within a select subset in the United States by Peppard and colleagues[7] also clearly showed the increasing prevalence of OSA. OSA has truly become a major entity, so much so that in 2013 the National Healthy Sleep Awareness Project was formed. As a national campaign, it was established by a cooperative agreement between the Centers for Disease Control and Prevention and the American Academy of Sleep Medicine to help with sleep health awareness.

One of the major epidemiologic changes that have likely caused OSA rates to increase is the nationwide obesity epidemic, with rates of obesity increasing from 15% in 1990[8] to 36% in 2012.[9] The increase in overweight and obese adults and children has fueled a significant increase in their medical comorbidities. Current prevalence numbers for OSA are in the realm of 36.1% in men and 11.4% in women ranging from 30 to 49 years of age. In the older subset, the author noted 60.6% in men and 36.9% in women between 50 and 70 years of age.[7] These rates vary by study, but the literature does support an overall increase in the past decade.

## ECONOMIC IMPACT OF OBSTRUCTIVE SLEEP APNEA

With the increasing prevalence of OSA, the economic impact of OSA cannot be overstressed. The impact can be broken down several ways. First, the cost directly to patients has been evaluated in the past. In 1999, Kapur and colleagues[10] showed that the annual health care cost to patients directly the year before diagnosis of OSA was $1336 higher and almost double overall when compared with age- and sex-matched controls without OSA. This study went on to estimate that cost of the medical comorbidities alone in 1999 to be $3.4 billion in the United States. To date, multiple studies have shown a large increase in health care utilization in patients with OSA as well.[11,12]

Not only are there direct costs to health care when considering OSA as a clinical entity but we must also consider the workday's lost and inherent disability that OSA may cause. Data from the Integrated Benefits Institute shows individuals with sleep disturbances are also less likely to be productive at work, with an average of 7.9 more absence days and 7.5 more present days.[13] There are also good data that shows patients with OSA and excessive daytime sleepiness are at higher risk of both recent work disability and longer-term work duty modification.[14] These effects on work days lost and productivity for patients with OSA are just another marker of the disease's costs.

## RISK FACTOR FOR OTHER CONDITIONS

As a health care provider, the largest cost of OSA is the increased comorbid conditions that our patients must struggle with. OSA was noted to be an independent risk factor for stroke and subsequent associated death.[15] It has also been shown to be a risk factor for fatal and nonfatal cardiovascular events.[16] Punjabi and colleagues[17] also showed that sleep-disordered breathing is independently associated with glucose intolerance and insulin resistance. The list of other conditions that OSA predisposes patients for includes but is not limited to hypertension, increased inflammatory markers, early signs of atherosclerosis, and in select groups even mild cognitive impairment.[18–20]

## PERIOPERATIVE COMPLICATIONS

OSA also inherently increases the risk of perioperative complications, and this does not apply solely on airway surgeries. Vasu and colleagues[21] performed a systematic review showing that patients with OSA had multiple different increased perioperative complications. In their review, they detailed several specific studies, including Gupta and colleagues[22] study that showed a more than a double increase in perioperative complications for patients with OSA undergoing orthopedic procedures and the Kaw and colleagues[23] study that showed increased rates of encephalopathy, postoperative infections and intensive-care-unit stay in cardiac surgery patients with OSA. The increased perioperative complications are likely due to opioids and their associated sedative effects combined with postanesthesia rapid-eye-movement sleep rebound causing a worsening of sleep apnea. These studies show the importance of identifying patients with OSA and optimizing their treatment early on.

In summary, OSA is a detrimental disease process that has direct implications on individual and society health status. The need for evidence-based and targeted treatment is clear, and the subsequent articles will help delineate the various treatment options.

## REFERENCES

1. Burwell CS. Extreme obesity associated with alveolar hypoventilation: a pickwickian syndrome. Am J Med 1956;21:811–8.
2. Gastaut H, Tassinari CA, Duron B. Polygraphic study of the episodic diurnal and nocturnal (hypnic and respiratory) manifestations of the Pickwick syndrome. Brain Res 1966;1(2):167–86.
3. Broadbent WH. Cheyne-Stokes' respiration in cerebral hemorrhage. Lancet 1877:307–9
4. Caton R. Clinical Society of London. Narcolepsy. BMJ. 18891358–35.
5. Lavie P. Nothing new under the moon. Historical accounts of sleep apnea syndrome. Arch Intern Med 1984;144(10):2025–8.
6. Franklin KA, Linderberg E. Obstructive sleep apnea is a common disorder in the population-a review on the epidemiology of sleep apnea. Thorac Dis 2015;7(8): 1311–22.
7. Peppard PE, Young T, Barnet JH, et al. Increased prevalence of sleep-disordered breathing in adults. Am J Epidemiol 2013;177(9):1006–14.
8. Centers for Disease Control and Prevention. Overweight and obesity: adult obesity facts.
9. Flegal KM, Carroll MD, Kit BK, et al. Prevalence of obesity and trends in the distribution of body mass index among US adults, 1999-2010. JAMA 2012;307: 491–7.
10. Kapur V, Blough DK, Sanblom RE, et al. The medical cost of undiagnosed sleep apnea. Sleep 1999;22:749–55.
11. Kapur VK, Redline S, Nieto FJ, et al. The relationship between chronically disrupted sleep and healthcare use. Sleep 2002;25:289–96.
12. Tarasiuka A, Reuvenib H. The economic impact of obstructive sleep apnea. Curr Opin Pulm Med 2013;19(6):639–44.
13. Integrated Benefits Institute. Analysis of HPQ/HPQ-Select self-report database.
14. Omachi TA, Claman DM, Blanc PD, et al. Obstructive sleep apnea: a risk factor for work disability. Sleep 2009;32(6):791–8.

15. Yaggi HK, Concato J, Kernan WN, et al. Obstructive sleep apnea as a risk factor for stroke and death. N Engl J Med 2005;353:2034–41.

16. Marin JM, Carrizo SJ, Vincente E, et al. Long-term cardiovascular outcomes in men with obstructive sleep apnoea-hypopnoea with or without treatment with continuous positive airway pressure: an observational study. Lancet 2005;365: 1046–53.

17. Punjabi NM, Sorkin JD, Katzel LI, et al. Sleep-disordered breathing and insulin resistance in middle-aged and overweight men. Am J Respir Crit Care Med 2002;165:677–82.

18. Drager LF, Bortolotto LA, Lorenzi MC, et al. Early signs of atherosclerosis in obstructive sleep apnea. Am J Respir Crit Care Med 2005;172:613–8.

19. Drager LF, Lopes HF, Maki-Nunes C, et al. The impact of obstructive sleep apnea on metabolic and inflammatory markers in consecutive patients with metabolic syndrome. PLoS One 2010;5:e12065.

20. Nieto FJ, Young TB, Lind BK, et al. Association of sleep-disordered breathing, sleep apnea, and hypertension in a large community-based study. Sleep Heart Health Study. JAMA 2000;283:1829–36.

21. Vasu TS, Grewal R, Doghramji K. Obstructive sleep apnea syndrome and perioperative complications: a systematic review of the literature. J Clin Sleep Med 2012;8(2):199–207.

22. Gupta RM, Parvizi J, Hanssen AD, et al. Postoperative complications in patients with obstructive sleep apnea syndrome undergoing hip or knee replacement: a case-control study. Mayo Clin Proc 2001;76:897–905.

23. Kaw R, Golish J, Ghamande S, et al. Incremental risk of obstructive sleep apnea on cardiac surgical outcomes. J Cardiovasc Surg (Torino) 2006;47:683–9.

# How to Evaluate a Diagnostic Sleep Study Report

Lee Shangold, MD

## KEYWORDS

- Diagnostic sleep study report • Obstructive sleep apnea • Sleep disorder

## KEY POINTS

- All in-laboratory sleep study reports should include sleep architecture, respiratory summary, periodic limb movements, sleep fragmentation and electrocardiography.
- Knowing what information to look for in all of these categories allows clinicians to treat patients with obstructive sleep apnea in a thoughtful and comprehensive way.
- Home sleep testing does not give as much information as an in-laboratory sleep study, but there are still some patients in whom a home sleep test may be more appropriate.

---

Otolaryngologists are frequently called upon to treat patients with obstructive sleep apnea (OSA). One of the most important tools we have to help us decide what treatment options, if any, are in the best interest of our patients is the sleep study.

A sleep study is a test that measures certain parameters to determine, among other things, a patient's degree of OSA. It can be used diagnostically or it can be used to measure a response to treatment, such as after surgery or with an oral appliance in place. A sleep study can be performed in a sleep lab or at home. It is usually performed at night. However, it is sometimes done during the day in patients, such as shift workers, who generally work at night and sleep during the day.

A sleep study can also be used as a therapeutic procedure in an attempt to treat a patient with OSA. This study can take the form of a continuous positive airway pressure (CPAP), bilevel positive airway pressure (BPAP), or adaptive servoventilation (ASV) titration. CPAP and BPAP titrations are performed to treat OSA, whereas an ASV titration is used in patients with central or complex sleep apnea.[1,2] In general, whichever modality is used, low pressure is used at the beginning of the study. The pressure is then slowly advanced, in response to respiratory events and snoring, until the optimal pressure setting is identified.

A therapeutic oral appliance titration can also be performed in the laboratory. During this study, the mandible is protruded by advancing the oral appliance in response to

---

ENT and Allergy Associates, 1500 Route 112, Port Jefferson Station, NY 11776, USA
*E-mail address:* Lshangold@entandallergy.com

Otolaryngol Clin N Am 49 (2016) 1307–1329
http://dx.doi.org/10.1016/j.otc.2016.07.003
0030-6665/16/© 2016 Elsevier Inc. All rights reserved.

**oto.theclinics.com**

events, similar to a positive airway pressure (PAP) titration, within parameters set by the titrating physician/dentist prior to the study.[3]

There are other studies that are performed in a sleep lab. These studies include a multiple sleep latency test (MSLT) and a maintenance of wakefulness test (MWT).[4] The MSLT is used to assess someone's ability to fall asleep in an attempt to quantify hypersomnolence as well as to identify patients with narcolepsy. It entails 4 to 5 nap periods on the day following a full night diagnostic sleep study. An MWT is used to measure a patient's ability to maintain wakefulness. This test takes place during the day and consists of four 40-minute trials during which the patient sits up in bed with instructions to sit still and remain awake for as long as possible. It is frequently used for patients whose work, and ability to stay awake, may affect public safety.

The gold standard diagnostic sleep study is an in-laboratory polysomnography. Understanding the information that can be gleaned from an in-laboratory sleep study not only allows clinicians to treat patients with OSA but also allows home sleep apnea tests (HSATs) to be put in perspective.

When reviewing a sleep study with a patient in the office, it is easy to look at the apnea-hypopnea index (AHI) and/or respiratory disturbance index (RDI) and decide on treatment options. However, there is more information on a sleep study report than just the AHI/RDI. If clinicians know what information to look for on a sleep study report, it allows a more comprehensive and effective treatment plan for our patients with OSA.

How a sleep study report looks is predicated on what software was used to create it. Thus, sleep studies from 2 different sleep labs may look very different. However, if clinicians understand what categories to look for in a sleep study report, and what information is important within each category, it becomes easy to get the most information out of any given report. If most of the sleep studies assessed by a physician come from 1 laboratory, it is simple, within a short period of time, to be able to quickly peruse a study for what information is important and relevant.

Before looking at what general categories make up a sleep study report, it is helpful to look at what information is collected during a sleep study and how this information is presented.

After patients check in at the sleep lab, they are brought to a private room. The sleep lab technician then hooks up the patient by attaching all of the appropriate leads. The patient is then instructed to go to sleep. During the course of the night, data are collected from all of the leads. If a lead falls off, the technician sees this on a computer monitor in a separate monitoring room and goes back into the patient's room to reattach the lead. After the patient leaves the laboratory, the collected data are then scored by a sleep technologist. The sleep technologist puts in the stages of sleep and marks the events. Subsequently, this scored study is then interpreted by a sleep physician who looks at all of the scored data and restages sleep/wakefulness and overscores events as deemed necessary.

It is beyond the scope of this article to teach readers how to score and interpret the raw data on a sleep study, but it will be easier for readers to look at a sleep study report if they have a visual of what is recorded during the course of a study night.

The leads used during an in-laboratory diagnostic sleep study are standardized.[5] Each lead contributes to the overall picture that develops during the course of a study. The leads that are represented on the top half of sleep study raw data help clinicians to determine whether someone is awake or asleep. The leads represented on the bottom half of the page/screen generally provide information about events, including respiratory events, limb movements, and cardiac events (**Fig. 1**).

The top half of a sleep study screen includes 2 electrooculography (EOG), or eye, leads; 6 electroencephalography (EEG) leads; and a chin electromyography (EMG)

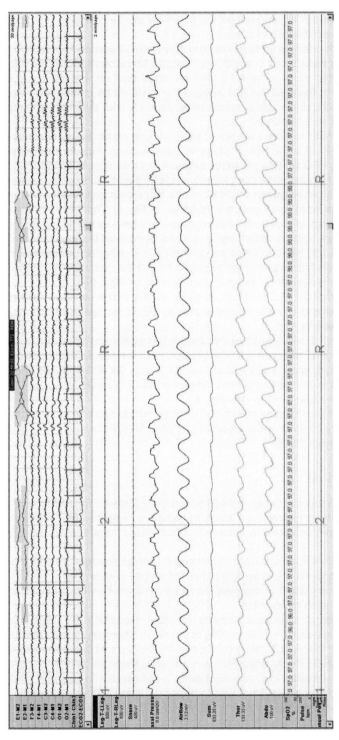

**Fig. 1.** Full screen of a sleep study. The top half is viewed in a 30-second window and the bottom half in a 2-minute window. The leads from top to bottom include 2 eye movement leads, 6 electroencephalography (EEG) leads, a chin electromyography (EMG) leads, electrocardiography (ECG) lead, 2 leg leads, snore microphone, nasal pressure, airflow, the sum of the effort belts, thoracic and abdominal effort belts, pulse oximetry, pulse, and body position.

lead. As stated earlier, taken together, these leads have definable findings that help clinicians determine not only whether the patient is awake or asleep but, if asleep, what stage of sleep the patient is in.

In a sleep study, sleep is artificially broken down into 30-second epochs. Whatever stage of sleep, or wakefulness, constitutes most of a 30-second epoch is the stage the epoch gets scored as. If a patient's total recorded time on a sleep study is, for example, 5 hours, there will be 600 epochs that need to be staged. Five hours is 300 minutes. Each minute has 2 epochs of 30 seconds and, therefore, 300 minutes × 2 epochs/min = 600 epochs.

Findings that help to define stages of sleep include alpha waves encompassing greater than 50% of an epoch in stage W (wakefulness) (**Fig. 2**); low-amplitude, mixed-frequency EEG activity and alpha waves of less than 50% of an epoch in stage N1 (**Fig. 3**); sleep spindles and K complexes in stage N2 (**Fig. 4**); and delta waves in stage N3 (**Fig. 5**). Clearly, when asleep, the EOG, or eye, leads, help to determine whether the patient is in stage rapid eye movement (REM) sleep (**Fig. 6**). The figures in this article show typical findings in drowsiness before sleep onset and each stage of sleep. They are presented here, and visualized best on a sleep study, in a 30-second window.

The chin EMG also helps to stage sleep. There is a steady decrease in tone represented on the EMG from wakefulness to stages N1, N2, N3, and then into stage REM. This progression is evident on the lowest line (green) on **Figs. 2–6**.

Keep in mind that the EEG montage, or configuration, that is used for sleep studies is not as comprehensive as the montage used for EEGs that are used specifically to assess seizure activity.

The bottom half of the page generally includes nasal pressure and airflow readings, chest and abdominal effort belt leads, a microphone to record snoring, body position sensor, electrocardiography (ECG), and 2 leg EMG leads. All of these leads are generally best viewed in a 2-minute screen, other than the ECG lead, which is easier to analyze in a 30-second window (see **Fig. 1**).

In general, there are 5 categories to look for in a sleep study: sleep architecture, respiratory summary, periodic limb movements, arousal analysis or sleep fragmentation, and cardiac analysis (ECG).

## SLEEP ARCHITECTURE

In life, there are 3 states of being: wakefulness, non-REM sleep, and REM sleep. When everything is working well, these 3 states of being are separate and distinct. People flow smoothly from one state to another in a fairly standard pattern during a typical 24-hour period.

Sleep architecture is the basic structural organization and pattern of sleep. It is what happens with respect to the order and pattern of staging of sleep during the course of the night. One component of the sleep architecture is what percentage of the night people spend in each sleep stage.

As stated earlier, sleep is separated into non-REM sleep and REM sleep. In adults, non-REM sleep is usually ~75% to 80% of the night, whereas stage REM is usually ~20% to 25% of the night.[6] Until recently, non-REM sleep was separated into stages 1, 2, 3, and 4. In 2008, the American Academy of Sleep Medicine (AASM) discontinued the use of stage 4 sleep. Now, non-REM sleep is separated into stages N1, N2, and N3. Stage N3 encompasses what used to be stages 3 and 4.[5]

Normal sleep architecture changes with age. Not only do newborns spend much more time sleeping during a 24-hour period than adults, but they spend ~50% of their sleep in stage REM or active sleep. Stage N3 sleep slowly decreases with age.

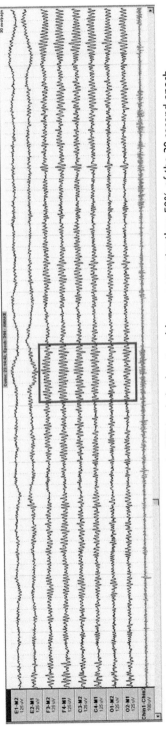

**Fig. 2.** Drowsy (before sleep onset) alpha waves, seen in EEG leads (*red rectangle*), occupy greater than 50% of the 30-second epoch.

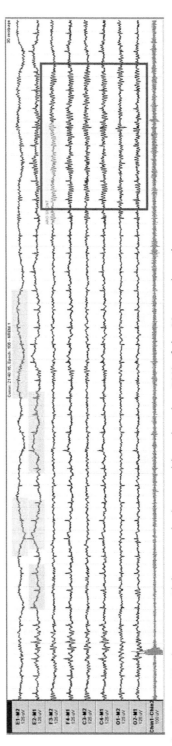

**Fig. 3.** Stage N1, sleep onset. Alpha waves (*red rectangle*) are less than 50% of the 30-second epoch.

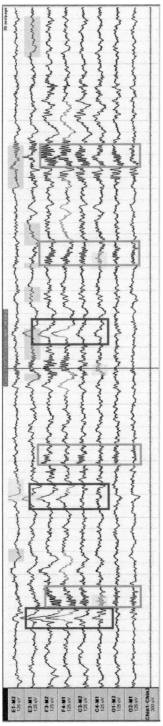

**Fig. 4.** Stage N2: K complexes (*red rectangles*) and sleep spindles (*green rectangles*).

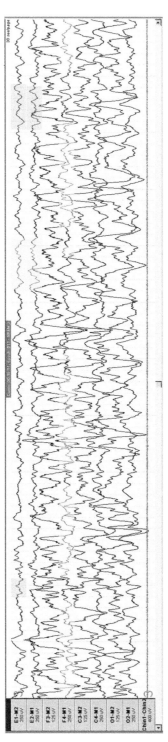

**Fig. 5.** Stage N3 or slow-wave sleep: numerous delta waves.

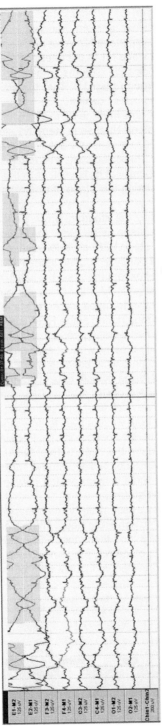

**Fig. 6.** Stage REM. Note REMs on the top 2 lines and low tone on chin EMG on the bottom line.

Stage N1 sleep is light or drowsy sleep with a very low arousal threshold. It is frequently the interface between wakefulness and the deeper stages of sleep. It is nonrestorative. When falling asleep at night, people generally go from wakefulness, briefly into stage N1, and then into stage N2. After awakenings at night, people sometimes again transition through stage N1 to the deeper stages of sleep. Some patients with very severe OSA, or significantly disrupted sleep for any reason, have frequent arousals and then transition through stage N1. They therefore have a much higher percentage of stage N1 than is normal or desired.

Adults generally spend more time in stage N2 than any other stage of sleep. There is a higher arousal threshold in stage N2 than in stage N1 sleep.

Stage N3, or slow-wave sleep, is generally considered to be the deepest stage of sleep and the most restorative. Physiologically, it is a very stable stage to be in. During this stage, the heart rate is generally at its lowest, as is the blood pressure. Sleep apnea events are less frequent during this stage of sleep than in any other sleep stage because of its stability.

Stage REM sleep is generally the stage in which people dream. Physiologically, several things happen during stage REM. First, the brain is very active. The brain uses as much glucose during stage REM as it does when awake.[7]

Second, people are in effect paralyzed during stage REM. People lose muscle tone in all of the muscles of the body except the eyes, the heart, and the diaphragm. If people had muscle tone during stage REM, they could get out of bed and act out their dreams. It is, therefore, protective to be paralyzed in stage REM.

The inability to lose muscle tone during stage REM is seen in an entity called REM Behavior Disorder. This entity can be dangerous to the patient, and to those around the patient. Patients act out their dreams without an awareness of the consequences. This condition is seen most commonly in patients with Parkinson's disease.

In contrast, the downside of losing muscle tone in stage REM is that many patients with OSA tend to have a higher AHI or RDI in stage REM than in non-REM sleep. Less muscle tone leads to more airway collapse, and therefore, more respiratory events.

Adults with normal sleep go from wakefulness to drowsiness to non-REM sleep. After ~80 to 110 minutes, the first REM period occurs. People generally go through 4 to 6 non-REM to REM cycles during the night before awakening in the morning. This sequence can be seen most easily on a sleep study report by looking at the hypnogram. The hypnogram is an overall view or gestalt of what transpired in the course of a night with respect to sleep staging.

The hypnogram in Fig. 7 shows essentially normal sleep architecture. It shows a patient going from wakefulness into non-REM sleep. The patient then transitions through stage N2 and then into stage N3, and then stage REM. This patient has 6 non-REM/REM cycles. Slow-wave sleep, stage N3, predominates in the first third of the night, whereas stage REM is more prevalent in the last third of the night.

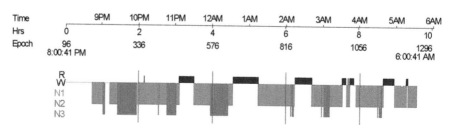

**Fig. 7.** Hypnogram of essentially normal sleep architecture (*gray line* is wakefulness, *yellow* is stage N1, *green* is stage N2, *blue* is stage N3 and *red* is stage REM).

The hypnogram in **Fig. 8** is representative of a patient with very severe OSA. Note how he cannot stay in the deeper stages of sleep and has frequent arousals with reentry to sleep through Stage N1 (yellow). After the hypnogram, the author looks at a table that shows what percentage of the night was spent in each stage of sleep and compares this with normal values.

The total sleep time (TST) is the amount of time during the night that the patient was asleep, as verified by EEG.

Sleep efficiency is the percentage of the night, from the time the sleep technician says "Lights out, go to sleep" until the lights are turned on in the morning, that the patient was actually sleeping. Normal sleep efficiency is greater than 85%. Keep in mind that the patient is sleeping in a strange place and is attached to many wires, which may decrease the patient's sleep efficiency artificially. This is especially true during the patient's first sleep study secondary to what is called "first-night effect" in the sleep lab.[8]

The sleep latency shows how long it took for the patient to get into the first epoch of sleep from the time the technician says, "Lights out, go to sleep." Normal sleep latency is less than 30 minutes. Again, keep in mind that a decreased sleep efficiency and an increased sleep latency may be secondary to the environment in which the patient is sleeping in.

In contrast, a high sleep efficiency (eg, 98%) with a low sleep latency (eg, 2 minutes), in this kind of environment, may be secondary to significant hypersomnolence; the patient is so tired that they can fall asleep anywhere, anytime, under any circumstances.

The author frequently sees patients who are dragged into the office by their bed partners for snoring, and possible sleep apnea. The patient may deny that they have any sleep issues because they can fall asleep anywhere as soon as their head hits the pillow. Here is an opportunity to explain to them that this is not normal. A normal sleep latency is 5 to 30 minutes, not 30 seconds.

Another latency that is very important is the REM latency. This is how long it takes a person to progress from the first epoch of sleep to the first epoch of stage REM sleep. Normal REM latency is 80 to 110 minutes. A very short REM latency, such as 5 minutes, can be pathologic. It suggests, but is not pathognomonic for, the possibility of narcolepsy.

Narcolepsy is the intermingling of wakefulness and stage REM sleep. The symptom of cataplexy is pathognomonic for narcolepsy but is only seen in ~50% of patients with narcolepsy. Cataplexy is a sudden attack of muscle weakness that is usually triggered by strong emotion (laughing more commonly than crying).

As can be seen above, there is a lot of useful information that can be obtained from understanding sleep architecture, both normal and abnormal, before even considering the respiratory summary.

## RESPIRATORY SUMMARY

The respiratory summary is the main section of a sleep study when the purpose is to establish whether the patient has sleep apnea and, if so, to what degree.

SLEEP STAGE SUMMARY

**Fig. 8.** Hypnogram of a patient with severe OSA (yellow is Stage N1, green is Stage N2, blue is Stage N3 and red is Stage REM).

To understand the respiratory summary, clinicians must first know the definitions of the terms that make up the all-important indices.[5] An apnea is defined as a decrease in the airflow by greater than 90% for at least 10 seconds (**Fig. 9**).

There are 2 definitions for a hypopnea, which is the most common respiratory event seen in the sleep lab. The definition that the AASM recommends is a decrease in nasal pressure by greater than 30% for at least 10 seconds with either a decrease in oxygen saturation by at least 3% or an arousal as determined by EEG (**Figs. 10** and **11**). The alternative definition that the Centers for Medicare and Medicaid Services require is a decrease in nasal pressure reading by greater than 30% for at least 10 seconds with a concomitant decrease in oxygen saturation by at least 4%. The relevance of these 2 definitions is that a patient with Medicare or Medicaid may have a lower AHI or RDI than a patient with commercial insurance despite having identical recordings. Therefore, it is important to know which criteria were used in the scoring of the study before treating the patient based on the study results.

The final respiratory event that can be included in degree of OSA is a respiratory effort–related arousal (RERA). This event does not meet the criteria for an apnea or hypopnea but nonetheless shows increased effort of breathing with a disruption in sleep. To be certain that there is an increase in respiratory effort before an arousal, patients need to have an esophageal probe in place, but very few patients would come to a sleep lab if this were the case. However, a RERA can be extrapolated from the typical data collected. There are signs of increased respiratory effort on the parameters that are measured, such as flattening of the nasal pressure curve.[9]

The 2 main indices that are used to measure degree of OSA are the AHI and the RDI:

AHI = (# of apneas + # of hypopneas)/TST

RDI = AHI + (# of RERAs/TST)

Some sleep labs report the AHI, some report the RDI, and some report both. The degree of OSA based on the AHI/RDI is as follows (**Table 1**).

Apneas can be divided into obstructive and central. An obstructive apnea, which is the more common type seen in the laboratory, is secondary to airway collapse with subsequent blockage of the upper airway during sleep. Central apneas are secondary to lack of signal from the brain to breathe. Central apneas are commonly seen in patients with congestive heart failure, people who are at high altitudes before acclimating, patients on narcotics, and patients with primary central sleep apnea (CSA).

Patients in the sleep lab have belts around the chest and abdomen. These are effort belts. During an obstructive event, there is a signal coming from the belts that, despite the patient not breathing, the patient is trying to breathe. During a central event there is no signal coming from the belts, so there is no inspiratory effort. This distinction is important because OSA and CSA may be treated differently.[1]

In addition to the overall AHI/RDI, the AHI/RDI is also reported by position and REM versus non-REM sleep, which may have a significant impact on the recommendations of treatment.

OSA is usually worse in the supine position than in a non-supine position. Therefore, it is important to assess the total AHI/RDI as well as the supine and non-supine AHI/RDI. This information reveals whether positioning therapy is a potential treatment option for the patient. Positioning therapy can be performed using appropriate T-shirts, wedges, and pillows that are designed for this purpose.

As stated previously, OSA is usually worse in stage REM than in non-REM sleep. Thus, it is important to assess the percentage of stage REM that the patient had during

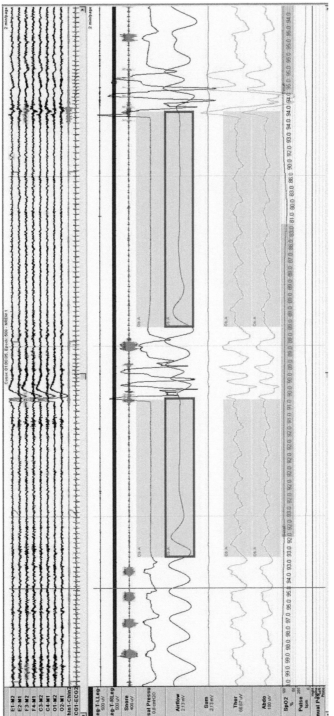

**Fig. 9.** Two obstructive apneas with a greater than 90% decrease in airflow (*red rectangles*) lasting longer than 10 seconds.

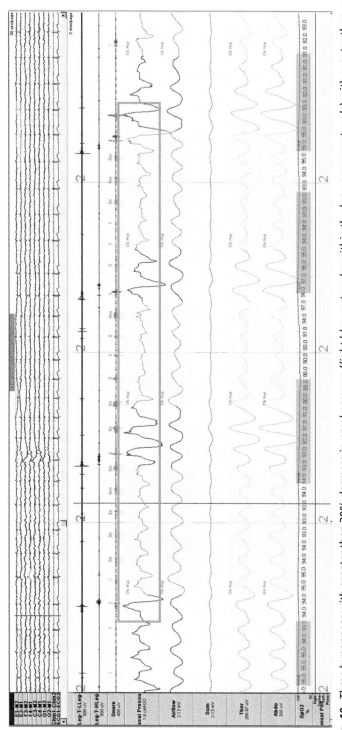

**Fig. 10.** Three hypopneas with greater than 30% decrease in nasal pressure (*light blue rectangles* within the *long green rectangle*) with greater than or equal to 3% decrease in oxygen saturation (*thin mauve rectangles* near the bottom of the page).

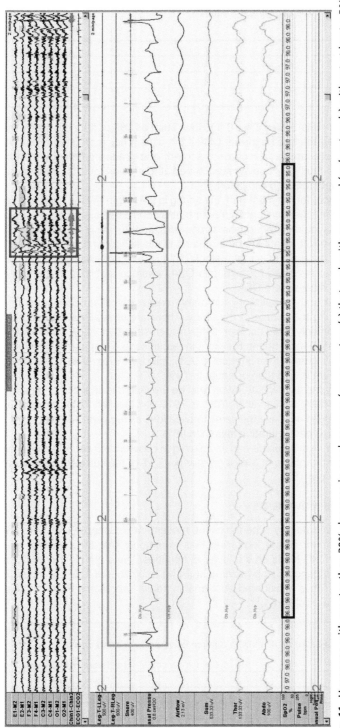

**Fig. 11.** Hypopnea with greater than 30% decrease in nasal pressure (*green rectangle*) that ends with an arousal (*red rectangle*) without at least a 3% decrease in oxygen saturation (*long black rectangle*).

| Table 1 | |
|---|---|
| Degree of OSA based on AHI/RDI in adults | |
| AHI/RDI (/h) | Degree of OSA |
| <5 | Essentially normal |
| 5–15 | Mild |
| 15–30 | Moderate |
| >30 | Severe |

the night (normal is 20%–25%). If it is low, such as 0% or 5%, this study may have underestimated the true degree of OSA if the patient has more stage REM at home.

Pediatric sleep apnea is recorded, scored, and graded differently than in adults (**Table 2**). End-tidal $CO_2$ is evaluated in pediatric studies, but not adult studies. It is used to evaluate for hypoventilation.[10]

The difference, for the most part, in scoring is the length of time needed to score an event and the number of events per hour that is considered significant. As opposed to the 10 seconds required for apneas, hypopneas, and RERAs in adults, with children an event is scored, if it meets the other criteria, if it lasts longer than 2 breaths.

In addition, the grading is much stricter in children. For example, an adult with an AHI of 14/h is considered to have mild OSA, whereas a child with this same AHI is considered to have severe OSA.

The last part of the respiratory summary to assess is what happens to the oxygen saturation during the course of the study. There are several ways to approach this. The most commonly listed number is the oxygen saturation nadir, which is the lowest oxygen saturation seen during the night in response to a respiratory event. In general terms, normal is greater than or equal to 90%, mild is 85% to 89%, moderate is 80% to 84%, and severe is less than or equal to 79%.

Another way the oxygen saturation may be presented is as a percentage of the TST from 90% to 100%, 80% to 89%, 70% to 79%, and less than 70%. Clearly, a fleeting nadir of 79% does not have the same implications as a patient who spent 10% of the night with an oxygen saturation less than 80%.

In addition, it may be presented as an oxygen desaturation index, which is either the number of desaturations of 3% or greater per TST or the number of desaturations of 4% or greater per TST.

## PERIODIC LIMB MOVEMENTS

The next broad category is periodic limb movements of sleep (PLMS). PLMS is a repetitive movement of the legs, and less commonly the arms, during sleep. It is measured by EMG leads on the lower extremities. There are clear criteria that need to be met for a periodic limb movement (PLM) to be scored.[5] A PLM index (PLMI) of greater than 15/h is considered abnormal in adults, whereas a PLMI of greater than 5/h is abnormal in children.[11]

| Table 2 | |
|---|---|
| Degree of OSA based on AHI/RDI in children less than 18 years of age | |
| AHI/RDI (/h) | Degree of OSA (<18 y of Age) |
| <1 | Essentially normal |
| 1–5 | Mild |
| 5–10 | Moderate |
| >10 | Severe |

PLMs may or may not be associated with an EEG arousal (**Fig. 12**). They can disrupt sleep and contribute to excessive daytime sleepiness (EDS); for example, a patient who snores and has significant EDS. A sleep study is obtained that reveals an RDI of ∼2/h and a PLMI of greater than 50/h. It may be the PLMs that are contributing to the EDS.

Patients are considered to have PLM disorder (PLMD) if they have an increased PLMI and some daytime consequence, such as EDS, that is not secondary to some other cause. Patients who have an increased PLMI but no sequelae secondary to this are not considered to have PLMD.

PLMS is thought to be related to restless legs syndrome (RLS). RLS is a diagnosis made solely by history. The diagnosis of PLM is made by a sleep study. RLS is a sensory disorder; that is, it can be felt. PLMD is a motor disorder. Bed partners of patients with PLMS may say that they kick their legs during sleep. More than 80% of patients with RLS have an increased PLMI on a sleep study. In contrast, less than 30% of patients with PLMS have RLS.[12]

RLS and PLMs share the same pathophysiology and often respond to the same medication. The cause remains unclear but is most likely related to dopaminergic systems and brain iron metabolism. There are some potentially controllable exacerbating factors, including sleep deprivation, caffeine, selective serotonin reuptake inhibitors, alcohol, nicotine, and iron deficiency. They are seen more commonly in patients who are pregnant or have renal failure, myelopathy, diabetes, or Parkinson disease. If the patient has an increased PLMI, blood work for possible contributing factors should be considered, including serum ferritin, complete blood count , blood urea nitrogen/creatinine levels, thyroid function tests (TFTs), folate level, and vitamin $B_{12}$ level.

## SLEEP FRAGMENTATION

The fourth major category to be assessed on a sleep study report is sleep fragmentation. Frequently, the driving force behind a sleep evaluation is the symptom of EDS. This category may help to determine the underlying cause for this particular symptom.

As stated previously, in-laboratory sleep studies use an EEG montage to show when a patient is awake versus asleep and, if asleep, what stage of sleep the patient is in. In addition, the EEG identifies arousals from sleep. Every arousal gets marked and assigned a cause, if known. Clinicians want to know the cause of the arousals so that they can evaluate what is disrupting the patient's sleep.

Some arousals occur at the end of an apnea, hypopnea, or RERA (obviously, there cannot be a respiratory effort–related arousal without an arousal). These arousals are all clearly respiratory related secondary to sleep disordered breathing (SDB). Some arousals occur after a limb movement, and these are called limb movement arousals. If the cause of an arousal is not clear, it is categorized as a spontaneous arousal.

Spontaneous arousals have several different possible causes, which are not usually obvious from the sleep study. Spontaneous arousals may be secondary to hypervigilance from sleeping in a strange place, and being attached to multiple leads with a camera watching the person sleeping. Spontaneous arousals frequently are secondary to any form of pain, such as fibromyalgia or chronic back pain.

In a sleep study report, there is a section for arousals. It may be called Sleep Arousals or Sleep Fragmentation. There is a respiratory arousal index, a PLM arousal index, a spontaneous arousal index, and a total arousal index, and these are important in evaluating patients who have EDS that is not explained by OSA.

Also, keep in mind that there are causes of EDS other than SDB. Probably the most common cause for EDS is insufficient sleep. Average adults need ∼7.5 hours of sleep to function optimally. Teenagers need ∼9 hours of sleep. Causes for EDS other than

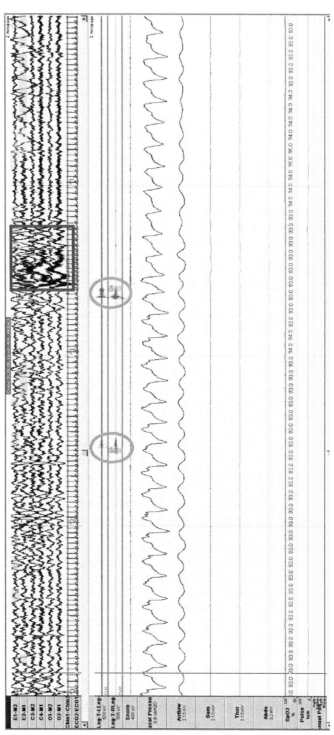

**Fig. 12.** Periodic limb movements (*green ovals*), one of which has an associated arousal (*red rectangle*), with normal nasal pressure, airflow, and pulse oximetry readings.

insufficient sleep, SDB, and PLM include, but are not limited to, medication side effect, mood disorder (especially depression), RLS, circadian rhythm disorders, insomnia, narcolepsy, and idiopathic hypersomnia. Tools to help clinicians make the correct diagnosis for EDS include comprehensive sleep history, sleep study, 2-week sleep log, Beck Depression Inventory, and MSLT.

## CARDIAC ANALYSIS

An additional category on an in-laboratory sleep study is the cardiac analysis, which is usually just a sentence or two about the ECG reading during the course of the night. Having the ECG in a sleep study is akin to having a Holter monitor.

Untreated moderate and severe OSA are independent risk factors for, among other things, hypertension and myocardial infarction. In some patients with significant OSA, the first sign of resultant cardiac disorder is ECG abnormalities seen during a sleep study (**Fig. 13**). Such things as multifocal premature ventricular contractions or heart block (other than Wenckebach) can be signs of significant cardiac disease that needs to be addressed in a timely fashion, in addition to the OSA.

## HOME SLEEP APNEA TESTING

To this point, this article has been about in-laboratory sleep study reports. HSATs have become prevalent over the last several years, partially because some patients tolerate an HSAT better, but mostly because it is dictated by some insurance companies in an attempt to save money. In the long run, this may not be true.[13]

**Table 3** shows the parameters that are measured in all in-laboratory studies compared with what is measured with HSATs.

This process can be taken a step further. **Table 4** shows which of the 5 main categories discussed in this article can be seen in HSATs. As stated previously, the respiratory summary is the basis of sleep testing and is what is ultimately used to assess someone's degree of OSA.

Also keep in mind that on in-laboratory sleep study reports, the all-important indices, AHI, RDI, and PLMI, use TST as the denominator in their equations. For example:

$$AHI = \frac{(\text{total \# of apneas}) + (\text{total \# of hypopneas})}{(\text{total sleep time})}$$

HSAT devices either use total recorded time or some surrogate measure for sleep, such as actigraphy, for the denominator. If the patient has a low sleep efficiency, total recorded time, as the denominator, gives a falsely low index. In contrast, actigraphy is a reasonable measure of sleep in that it records movement; for example, of the wrist. The wrist movement is generally different whether a person is awake or asleep.

There are advantages and disadvantages of both in-laboratory tests and HSATs. The advantages of in-laboratory studies include that there are consistent, easily reviewable data; that clinicians can diagnose and treat OSA in a single split-night sleep study in which the first half of the night is a diagnostic portion and the second half is a therapeutic PAP titration; and that disorders other than OSA can be identified. Such disorders include seizures, PLMs, and malignant arrhythmias.

The advantages of home sleep studies include potential cost savings; the comfort and convenience of patients sleeping in their own homes; and fewer leads attached and, therefore, possibly a more typical night sleep than might be seen in the laboratory.

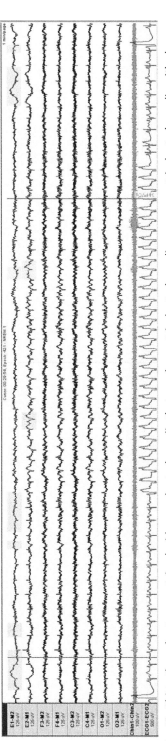

**Fig. 13.** Thirty-three–beat nonsustained wide complex tachycardia that may be ventricular tachycardia or supraventricular tachycardia with aberrancy. Cardiology evaluation for structural heart disease should be pursued.

**Table 3**
**In-laboratory versus HST parameters measured**

| In-laboratory Parameters Measured | HST Parameters Measured |
| --- | --- |
| Airflow: nasal/oral | Airflow: nasal/oral or arterial tone[a] |
| Pulse oximetry | Pulse oximetry[a] |
| Effort: thoracic/abdominal | Effort[b] |
| Body position | Body position[b] |
| ECG | ECG (almost all include pulse)[c] |
| Leg movements | Leg movements[c] |
| Eye movements | Eye movements[c] |
| EEG | EEG[c] |
| EMG: chin | EMG: chin[c] |

[a] HSAT parameters that are always measured.
[b] HSAT parameters that are usually measured.
[c] HSAT parameters that are infrequently measured.

## SUMMARY

When seeing a patient in the office to review the results of a sleep study, I first spend a minute looking at the study before walking into the examination room. I want to know what transpired during the night the patient spent in the sleep lab. In addition, I want to formulate what options to present to the patient to manage any sleep-related issues that the patient may have.

It is easy to look at the AHI/RDI, walk into the examination room, and explain that the patient has a certain degree of OSA and what the treatment options are. Clinicians may be confronted with a patient who has slept in the sleep lab for as little as 35 minutes all night. The patient may ask how a treatment plan can be formulated if the patient did not sleep. If the clinician had checked the TST (35 minutes) and sleep efficiency (10%), the clinician would have started the conversation with a phrase such as, "I see you had a poor night's sleep in the lab. Please tell me this is not a typical night's sleep for you." Instead of losing the patient's confidence, the clinician now has the patient's attention. First-night effect in the sleep lab can be explained to the patient and other options presented, including an HSAT.

Another example of using all of the information on a sleep study to treat the patient in a thoughtful fashion is as follows. A 62-year-old man presented to the laboratory with a

**Table 4**
**Comparison of what is included in an in-laboratory versus HST reports**

| In-laboratory Study Reports | HST Reports |
| --- | --- |
| Respiratory summary | Respiratory summary[a] |
| Sleep architecture | Sleep architecture[b] |
| ECG | ECG (almost all include pulse)[c] |
| Periodic limb movements | Periodic limb movements[c] |
| Sleep fragmentation | Sleep fragmentation[c] |

[a] HSAT reports include category always.
[b] HSAT reports include category sometimes.
[c] HSAT reports include categories infrequently.

**Table 5**
**RDI totals in a patient with very positional OSA**

| | By Sleep Stage | | By Position | | |
| | NREM | REM | Supine | Non-supine | Total |
|---|---|---|---|---|---|
| Sleep Time (min) | 198.5 | 39.5 | 176.5 | 61.5 | 238.0 |
| Apnea | | | | | |
|   Obstructive | 11 | 21 | 32 | 0 | 32 |
|   Mixed | 4 | 1 | 5 | 0 | 5 |
|   Central | 47 | 2 | 48 | 1 | 49 |
| Total Apnea | 62 | 24 | 85 | 1 | 86 |
| Apnea Index | 18.7 | 36.5 | 28.9 | 1.0 | 21.7 |
| Hypopnea | 144 | 7 | 149 | 2 | 151 |
| Total Apneas and Hypopneas | 206 | 31 | 234 | 3 | 237 |
| AHI | 62.3 | 47.1 | 79.5 | 2.9 | 59.7 |
| Flow Limitation Events (RERA) | 2 | 0 | 1 | 1 | 2 |
| RDI | 62.9 | 47.1 | 79.8 | 3.9 | **60.3** |

*Abbreviation:* NREM, non–REM sleep.

history of snoring, witnessed apnea, EDS, and coronary artery disease (CAD). His sleep study revealed severe OSA with an overall RDI of 60.3/h (**Table 5**). After a titration, he was put on CPAP. He did not tolerate it.

On reevaluating the patient's original sleep study, he clearly had overall severe OSA, but it was exceedingly positional. He had a supine RDI of 79.8/h and a non-supine RDI of 3.9/h. Further history revealed that the patient rarely slept on his back at home. He felt obligated to sleep mostly supine while in the sleep lab secondary to all of the wires

**Table 6**
**Summary of how to evaluate sleep study report**

| | What to Look at in Sleep Study Report | Significance |
|---|---|---|
| 1 | AHI/RDI | Gives degree of OSA |
| 2 | TST/sleep efficiency/ hypnogram | Gives a sense of how well the patient slept |
| 3 | REM latency | Normal is 80–110 min; if exceedingly low (ie, <20 min), consider evaluation for narcolepsy |
| 4 | AHI/RDI in supine and non-supine positions | Consider positioning therapy if very positional |
| 5 | Percentage of stage REM | If none or low, total AHI/RDI may underestimate degree of OSA |
| 6 | Periodic limb movement index | If high, may be contributing to EDS, especially in patient with no, or well-treated, OSA |
| 7 | Total arousal index and breakdown of arousals | May help determine cause for EDS (ie, respiratory, limb movements, or spontaneous) |
| 8 | Oxygen saturation nadir and percentage <90% | Contributes to cardiovascular risk |
| 9 | EKG Summary | Identifies potentially unknown arrhythmias |

and the instructions of the sleep technician. He was intolerant of CPAP because it was set to his optimal pressure when he was in the supine position. When he slept non-supine at home, the pressure was not only too high, but possibly not even necessary. To achieve a comfort level for the patient sleeping non-supine at home, with a low RDI, an HSAT could be done and the patient instructed to sleep how he normally sleeps. This case provides another example of treating the patient based on all of the information that can be gleaned from a sleep study report.

**Table 6** lists what I look at on a sleep study report, and its significance, before discussing the study with the patient.

In conclusion, this article presents a pathway to comprehensively assess all of the information on a sleep study report in a way that allows clinicians to most effectively treat patients who have OSA, and other sleep disorders.

## REFERENCES

1. Aurora RN, Chowdhuri S, Ramar K, et al. The treatment of central sleep apnea syndromes in adults: practice parameters with an evidence-based literature review and meta-analyses. Sleep 2012;35(1):17–40.
2. Javaheri S, Brown LK, Randerath WJ. Clinical applications of adaptive servoventilation devices: part 2. Chest 2014;146(3):858–68.
3. Dieltjens M, Vanderveken OM, Heyning PH, et al. Current opinions and clinical practice in the titration of oral appliances in the treatment of sleep-disordered breathing. Sleep Med Rev 2012;16:177–85.
4. Standards of Practice Committee of the American Academy of Sleep Medicine. Practice parameters for clinical use of the multiple sleep latency test and the maintenance of wakefulness test. Sleep 2005;28(1):113–21.
5. Berry RB, Brooks R, Gamaldo CE, et al, American Academy of Sleep Medicine. The AASM manual for the scoring of sleep and associated events: rules, terminology and technical specifications, version 2.1. Darien (IL): AASM; 2014. Available at: www.aasmnet.org.
6. Carskadon MA, Dement WC. Normal human sleep: an overview. In: Kryger MH, Roth T, Dement WC, editors. Principles and practice of sleep medicine. New York: Elsevier Saunders; 2005. p. 13–23.
7. Maquet P, Dive D, Salmon E, et al. Cerebral glucose utilization during sleep-wake cycle in man determined by positron emission tomography and [18F]2-fluoro-2-deoxy-D-glucose method. Brain Res 1990;513(1):136–43.
8. Agnew HW, Webb WB, Williams RL. The first night effect: an EEG study of sleep. Psychophysiology 1966;2(3):263–7.
9. Ayappa I, Norman RG, Krieger AC, et al. Non-invasive detection of respiratory effort-related arousals by a nasal cannula/pressure transducer system. Sleep 2000;23(6):763–71.
10. Beck SE, Marcus CL. Pediatric polysomnography. Sleep Med Clin 2009;4(3): 393–406.
11. American Academy of Sleep Medicine. International classification of sleep disorders, 2nd edition: diagnostic and coding manual. Westchester (IL): American Academy of Sleep Medicine; 2005.
12. Allen RP, Earley CJ. Defining the phenotype of the restless legs syndrome (RLS) using age-of-symptom-onset. Sleep Med 2000;1:11–9.
13. Pietzsch JB, Garner A, Cipriano LE, et al. An integrated health-economic analysis of diagnostic and therapeutic strategies in the treatment of moderate-to-severe obstructive sleep apnea. Sleep 2011;34(6):695–709.

# Positive Airway Pressure Therapy for Obstructive Sleep Apnea

 CrossMark

Pnina Weiss, MD[a],*, Meir Kryger, MD, FRCPC[b]

## KEYWORDS

- Positive airway pressure therapy • Continuous positive airway pressure
- Bilevel positive airway pressure • Autotitrating positive airway pressure
- Average volume assured pressure support • Adaptive support ventilation
- Obstructive sleep apnea syndrome • Pressure relief

## KEY POINTS

- Positive airway pressure (PAP) is considered first-line therapy for moderate to severe obstructive sleep apnea syndrome (OSAS) and may also be considered for mild obstructive sleep apnea, particularly if it is symptomatic or there are concomitant cardiovascular disorders.
- Continuous positive airway pressure (CPAP) is the most common initial mode of therapy for OSAS; however, bilevel positive airway pressure (BPAP) may be considered in patients who are unresponsive or intolerant of CPAP or who have concomitant respiratory insufficiency and hypoventilation.
- CPAP and BPAP are used in the autotitrating mode to initiate treatment or to determine the optimal pressure for patients with moderate to severe OSAS who do not have significant comorbidities.
- Adaptive support ventilation (ASV) is considered in patients with OSAS and respiratory insufficiency with central apnea; periodic breathing, such as Cheyne-Stokes respiration, or complex apnea. It is, however, contraindicated in patients with chronic heart failure with reduced ejection fraction less than or equal to 45%.
- Comfort features, such as mask interfaces, heated humidification, pressure relief modes, and ramps, have been developed to improve adherence to PAP, which despite proven efficacy, is low.

P. Weiss has no commercial conflict of interest.

M. Kryger is the principle investigator of a trial examining the efficacy of remote monitoring of positive airway pressure devices in military veterans (sponsors Respironics, Resmed), and a trial examining the efficacy of mandibular advancement devices in military veterans who will not use positive airway pressure (sponsors, Somnomed, Resmed). He is a scientific advisor to Inspire Medical and Dymedix.

[a] Pediatric Respiratory Medicine and Medical Education, Yale University School of Medicine, 333 Cedar Street, New Haven, CT 06520, USA; [b] Pulmonary, Critical Care and Sleep Medicine, Yale School of Medicine, 333 Cedar Street, New Haven, CT 06520, USA

* Corresponding author.

*E-mail address:* pnina.weiss@yale.edu

## BACKGROUND

Positive airway pressure (PAP) has been used to treat obstructive sleep apnea syndrome (OSAS) for more than 30 years.[1] PAP prevents upper airway collapse: it functions as a pneumatic splint,[2] increasing the caliber of the upper airway and it also increases lung volumes, which provides tracheal traction.[3] PAP is considered first-line therapy for moderate to severe obstructive sleep apnea and may also be considered for mild obstructive sleep apnea, particularly if it is symptomatic or there are concomitant cardiovascular disorders.[4–6] The indications for PAP include apnea hypopnea index (AHI) or respiratory disturbance index greater than or equal to 15 events per hour or AHI or respiratory disturbance index between 5 and 14 events per hour associated with symptoms such as excessive daytime sleepiness, impaired neurocognitive function, mood disorders, insomnia or cardiovascular disease (eg, hypertension, ischemic heart disease, congestive heart failure, atrial fibrillation) or history of stroke. The use of PAP for OSAS improves respiratory disturbances,[7] daytime sleepiness,[8,9] cognitive impairment,[10] mood,[11] and quality of life[12]; reduces automobile accidents[13,14]; and improves cardiovascular sequela, such as systemic hypertension.[15–17] Treatment of OSAS with PAP is optimized by using a multidisciplinary approach including a sleep specialist, the referring physician, nurses, respiratory therapists, and the sleep technologist.

## POSITIVE AIRWAY PRESSURE DELIVERY SYSTEMS

PAP devices are air pumps (fan-driven or turbine systems) that draw in external, filtered air to deliver pressured airflow. The airflow is adjusted by changing the diameter of the pressure valve or turbine/fan speed. Over the years, PAP machines have become more quiet, compact, and portable.

PAP is delivered by a variety of interfaces: nasal, oronasal, and oral (ie, nasal mask, nasal pillows, oronasal [face] mask, oral mask, and oral mask with nasal pillows). The choice of optimal interface is important, because it may influence a patient's acceptance of PAP therapy and long-term compliance.[18] The most commonly used interfaces are the face and nasal masks. Nasal pillows[19] and oral masks[20] may be considered as alternatives if a patient cannot tolerate the nasal or face masks. Face masks may be considered when nasal obstruction or mouth breathing limit the effectiveness of the nasal mask or greater inspired relative humidity is desired.[21] Masks have been developed by manufacturers to maximize patient comfort, using softer cushions.

Most currently available PAP devices include digital software that keeps track of date and time of usage, and detects and measures apnea, hypopnea (AHI), snore, flow limitation, periodic breathing, air leaks and flow waveform. In essence, these devices can measure many of the respiratory parameters that are monitored during a polysomnogram (PSG). Without the extensive monitoring of the PSG, it is not possible to determine the sleep stage of the patient or to accurately assess some of the physiologic complications of the OSAS. However, devices have advanced to the point that they can use the measured respiratory parameters to provide feedback in a closed-loop system and to manipulate the output variables.

## MODES OF POSITIVE AIRWAY PRESSURE

Many of the modes of PAP used for OSAS have variations of pressure-support or pressure-controlled ventilation. A target pressure is set and the resultant tidal volumes depend on the level of inspiratory pressure, respiratory system compliance, airway (upper and lower) resistance, and tubing resistance. Tidal volumes increase with increases in the inspiratory pressure and respiratory compliance and decreases in airway and device tubing resistance. In contrast, tidal volumes decrease with decreases in inspiratory pressure and respiratory compliance and increases in airway or device tubing resistance.

## CONTINUOUS POSITIVE AIRWAY PRESSURE

Continuous PAP (CPAP) is the initial and most commonly used modality for OSAS. It refers to the delivery of a continuous level of PAP, which is similar to positive end-expiratory pressure. The patient initiates all breaths; no additional pressure is given to support the individual breaths. The optimal setting for PAP titration is determined in an accredited sleep center or laboratory during a titration study, or obtained by examining data from an autotitrating device. It is important for all PAP candidates to receive adequate education, hands-on demonstration, careful mask fitting, and acclimatization before the titration. The goal of titration is to eliminate obstructive-related events, such as apneas, hypopneas, respiratory effort-related arousals, and snoring.[22] The recommended minimum starting CPAP is 4 cm $H_2O$, although higher levels are used in patients with obesity or for retitration studies. The maximum CPAP usually is 15 cm $H_2O$ for children and 20 cm $H_2O$ for patients greater than or equal to 12 years. CPAP is increased in a stepwise fashion by at least 1 cm $H_2O$ if obstructive events are seen. Once the optimal CPAP is obtained, then a downtitration may be performed.

Goals of the PAP titration study are a respiratory disturbance index (total of apneas, hypopneas, and respiratory effort-related arousals) less than 5 per hour, sea level oxygen saturation as measured by pulse oximetry greater than 90%, and an acceptable air leak around the mask.[22] In addition, the airflow tracing should be normalized and snoring should be eliminated. Optimal titrations include elimination of obstructive events during supine rapid eye movement sleep without producing arousals or awakenings. The full-night PSG is the optimal approach for titration; however, for some adults split-night titration studies may be adequate.[4] The effectiveness of split-night studies for titration of CPAP in children less than or equal to 12 years has not been adequately studied.

## BILEVEL POSITIVE AIRWAY PRESSURE

Bilevel PAP (BPAP) without a backup rate is indicated for patients with OSAS who do not respond to or are intolerant of CPAP. BPAP with a backup rate is indicated for patients with OSAS and respiratory insufficiency with hypoventilation caused by restrictive lung disease (ie, thoracic insufficiency, neuromuscular disease), obesity hypoventilation syndrome, central apnea and obstructive lung disease, such as chronic obstructive pulmonary disease (COPD).

BPAP is effective in improving gas exchange in patients with obstructive and restrictive lung disease.[17] In patients with OSAS who do not have coexisting daytime respiratory disease, BPAP may be used when CPAP is inadequate or not tolerated by the patient.[17] It is not usually used as first-line therapy, because the device that delivers BPAP is more expensive than the CPAP machine. BPAP delivers a preset inspiratory PAP (IPAP) and expiratory PAP (EPAP). The tidal volume depends on the difference between the IPAP and the EPAP (delta P). Increases in the delta P usually increase minute ventilation and can improve alveolar ventilation. The device coordinates the breath with the patient's inspiratory effort; the pressure-supported breath is triggered by a change in the patient's inspiratory air flow or airway pressure. In BPAP, a backup rate can be set if the patient is at risk for central apnea. The recommended starting pressures for IPAP and EPAP are 8 H$_2$O and 4 cm H$_2$O, respectively. The recommended maximum IPAP is 20 cm H$_2$O for children and 30 cm H$_2$O for patients greater than or equal to 12 years old. The minimum delta P is usually set at 4 cm H$_2$O and the maximum at 10 cm H$_2$O. Of note, the abbreviation "BiPAP" is often used interchangeably with BPAP. However, BiPAP is a proprietary term that refers to BPAP delivered with a specific company's device (Philips Respironics).

The potential advantages of BPAP when compared with CPAP include active ventilation (rather than just pneumatic splinting), decreased mean airway pressure (which could lead to better tolerance of the therapy), less respiratory muscle fatigue, and faster resolution of respiratory acidosis. There are few studies that compare the effectiveness of BPAP with CPAP in OSAS in either adults or children. In adults with obesity hypoventilation, one study found that BPAP was no better than CPAP as measured by gas exchange, sleepiness, or adherence, but it was associated with better sleep quality and psychomotor vigilance performance.[23] However, in most other studies in adults[22,23] and children[24] without coexisting daytime respiratory disease, BPAP offered no advantage over CPAP in either efficacy or adherence when used as initial treatment. There are some data to support that it is an effective alternative in patients who are intolerant of or nonadherent to CPAP.[25,26] One potential disadvantage of BPAP is patient-device asynchrony, which can lead to discomfort and ineffective ventilation.

## AUTOTITRATING POSITIVE AIRWAY PRESSURE

Autotitrating mode PAP (APAP) is indicated for patients with OSAS, and patients with OSAS nonresponsive or intolerant of fixed PAP. CPAP and BPAP may be used in an auto-titrating mode, which uses feedback from the patient's respiratory monitoring to automatically adjust airway pressures.[27] Its potential advantages include using it for initial titration of airway pressures in place of PSG in a sleep laboratory[28] and to decrease the mean airway pressure, which could improve patient compliance. For autotitrating CPAP, an airway pressure is set. If there are greater than a preset number of obstructive events (for example two events in a 3-minute period), the pressure is automatically increased in a stepwise fashion to a predetermined maximum. Once the obstructive episodes have been eliminated, then a downtitration is performed. APAP devices in the self-adjusting mode may be used for home studies to initiate treatment and to determine the optimal pressure for patients with OSAS who do not have significant comorbidities (eg, congestive heart failure, COPD, central sleep apnea syndromes, or hypoventilation syndromes).[29] The use of autotitrating CPAP has been associated with small improvements in adherence and sleepiness when compared with fixed CPAP, the clinical significance of which remains unclear.[30] However, autotitrating CPAP may actually be less effective than fixed CPAP at reducing the cardiovascular sequela associated with OSAS because it may cause more sympathetic activation.[31,32]

Autotitrating BPAP works in a similar manner. Preset inspiratory and expiratory pressures are used. If the patient has a critical number of obstructive events, then the pressures automatically increase in a stepwise fashion. In some algorithms, if an obstructive apnea occurs, EPAP increases and if an obstructive hypopnea occurs, then IPAP increases. To maintain adequate minute ventilation, a minimum delta P (ie 4 cm H$_2$O) is set. In one study, autotitrating BPAP further improved ventilation and obstructive events in patients who were intolerant or unresponsive to CPAP[33]; however, it is unclear whether the improvement was caused by the BPAP or the autotitrating mode.

## COMFORT FEATURES

Variations in the pattern of airflow during PAP, such as pressure relief modes and ramps, have been developed to improve patient comfort and adherence. A pressure relief mode was developed for CPAP and BPAP, because inspiration and exhalation against high pressures can produce dyspnea. In this mode, gradual, instead of abrupt, changes are used to deliver airway pressure. For example, in pressure relief mode with CPAP, a small decrease in airway pressure accompanies the beginning of exhalation. Additional modifications soften the pressure transition from inhalation to exhalation. In BPAP with pressure relief, there is a decrease in airway pressure at the beginning of exhalation and softening of the pressure transition from inhalation to exhalation and exhalation to inhalation. Studies have not consistently demonstrated that pressure relief when added to CPAP improves adherence or patient outcomes.[34–36] BPAP with pressure relief was associated with better compliance than CPAP alone in patients previous noncompliant with CPAP[26]; however, it is unclear whether the improvement was caused by the pressure relief or BPAP. Device manufacturers have developed devices that are tailored for female patients; they include unique APAP algorithms and gender-specific masks. Another comfort feature is a ramp that is used with patients who require a more gradual increase in PAP. In this method, there is a slow, stepwise increase to target pressures in the beginning of the cycle (ie, for 0–45 minutes). Some devices may be set to shorten this ramp period if they detect obstructive events. Use of the ramp has not been demonstrated to improve patient adherence.

## AVERAGE VOLUME ASSURED PRESSURE SUPPORT

Average volume assured pressure support (AVAPS) is indicated for patients with OSAS and respiratory insufficiency with hypoventilation caused by restrictive lung disease (ie, thoracic insufficiency, neuromuscular disease), obesity hypoventilation syndrome and obstructive lung diseases, such as COPD.

Patients who have complicated underlying cardiopulmonary disease may require modes of PAP support that guarantee active ventilation. BPAP can be used with AVAPS. In this mode, the device usually adjusts the IPAP to maintain a target tidal volume. For example, if IPAP, EPAP, and tidal volume are set at 15 cm $H_2O$, 6 cm $H_2O$, and 300 mL, respectively, when the tidal volume falls below 300 mL, the IPAP would increase to 17 cm $H_2O$ (if increments of 2 cm $H_2O$ are set) until either a tidal volume of 300 mL or a preset maximum IPAP is achieved. A backup rate is usually set. Indications for the use of BPAP AVAPS include patients with obstructive sleep apnea and chronic respiratory failure (ie, COPD, neuromuscular disease, restrictive lung disease, obesity hypoventilation syndrome). Newer technology has added the ability for the device to titrate IPAP/EPAP when obstructive events are detected. In addition, the device can decrease the respiratory rate to ensure full exhalation (particularly important in patients with COPD). However, no study has documented the superiority of BPAP AVAPS over BPAP alone in OSAS.[37]

## ADAPTIVE SUPPORT VENTILATION

Adaptive support ventilation (ASV) is indicated for patients with OSAS and respiratory insufficiency with central apnea; periodic breathing, such as Cheyne-Stokes respiration; or complex apnea. It is contraindicated in patients with chronic heart failure with reduced ejection fraction less than or equal to 45%.

ASV is a ventilatory mode that provides dynamic adjustment of inspiratory pressure support. ASV continuously monitors minute ventilation and airflow and, on a breath-to-breath basis, increases or decreases the pressure support. This mode can also be combined with autotitrating BPAP and has a backup rate in the event of central apnea. This mode is particularly useful in patients who have irregular breathing patterns, such as complex central or mixed sleep apneas and Cheyne-Stokes respiration.[38,39] However, the use of ASV in patients with symptomatic chronic heart failure with reduced ejection fraction (left ventricular ejection fraction ≤45%) to treat moderate-severe central sleep apnea syndrome has been associated with an increase in cardiovascular mortality.[40]

## COMPLICATIONS OF POSITIVE AIRWAY PRESSURE

Most patients experience at least one, usually mild, side effect of PAP.[17,41,42] Side effects include mask discomfort, claustrophobia or a sense of suffocation, air leaks, skin abrasion/ulceration, dermatitis, conjunctivitis, headache, nasal stuffiness, sneezing, dry nose and mouth, and aerophagia.[17,41,42] Less common effects include tinnitus; otitis; sinusitis; and, rarely, pneumocephalus, pulmonary barotrauma, increased intraocular pressure, tympanic membrane rupture, and subcutaneous emphysema.[43,44] PAP therapy should be used with caution after neurosurgery, facial surgery, or trauma. Central apneas occur in 5% to 10% of patients with OSAS after initiation of PAP treatment.[45,46] They are usually transient and resolve within 2 months; however, some patients require a switch to a ventilatory mode with active ventilation, such as ASV.[47] Patients and their spouses may find the equipment intrusive, cumbersome, and noisy. Equipment malfunction can occur because of condensation of water in the tubing and inadequate maintenance or cleaning. Side effects may adversely impact patient adherence.

## POSITIVE AIRWAY PRESSURE ADHERENCE

Despite the proven efficacy of PAP in treating OSAS and its sequelae, adherence to therapy is low in adults and children, often less than 50%.[24,48–51] Adherence is often defined as greater than or equal to 4 hours of PAP usage for greater than or equal to 70% of the nights monitored. The goal is for the patient to use the PAP for 7 hours/night every night; it is possible that benefit is obtained even at lower levels of PAP usage.[52] However, Medicare in the United States only covers the equipment if adherence is documented after initiation of PAP therapy as defined by use of 4 or more hours per night on 70% of nights during a consecutive 30-day period anytime during the first 3 months of use.[53] Documentation of adherence to PAP therapy must be determined through direct download or visual inspection of usage data with written documentation provided in a report to be reviewed by the treating physician and included in the patient's medical record.

Patterns of usage are usually established in the first weeks following initiation of PAP therapy.[51,54] Many attempts have been made to improve patient adherence. Heated humidification is recommended to improve patient comfort.[55,56] It is important to optimize the comfort and fit of the mask interface and minimize air leak. Educational, supportive, and behavioral interventions have met with modest success.[57–60] Patients should be educated about the function and care of their equipment, the benefits of therapy, and the potential side effects and problems. PAP use should be objectively monitored to assess compliance.

Smart cards, modem, or World Wide Web–based methodology can be used to obtain data on patient usage and respiratory parameters. Intensive patient education and frequent health provider contact can improve patient adherence.[61,62] Interactive World Wide Web–based applications have been developed that deliver feedback to the patient on usage, mask fit, and number of obstructive events. Patients can access motivational and educational tools directly from smartphones, tablets, or computers.

## FOLLOW-UP

It is important to establish close follow-up of patients after initiation of PAP therapy. PAP usage should be objectively monitored, because patients tend to overestimate their use. Close communication with patients should be established in their first few weeks of use, so problems are promptly remediated.[61] For Medicare in the United States to continue coverage of PAP after the 3-month trial period, the treating physician must evaluate the patient face-to-face between 31 and 91 days after initiating therapy and must document compliance (by review of objective usage data) and clinical benefit (that the patient has improved on PAP).[53] Follow-up of patients should include assessment of several important outcomes: resolution of sleepiness, quality of life, patient and spousal satisfaction with treatment, adherence to therapy, avoidance of factors that worsen OSAS, adequate sleep amount and hygiene, and weight management.[6] After initial PAP setup, long-term follow-up should be established yearly and as needed to address problems. Remote monitoring can allow easy access to data and allow the device settings to be adjusted remotely. If there is inadequate resolution of symptoms after initiation of PAP, it is important to determine whether there is persistent OSAS caused by inadequate PAP (suboptimal pressures, mask airflow leak, equipment failure, or nonadherence) or whether the symptoms are caused by concomitant medical or psychiatric diseases or another sleep disorder. If PAP adherence is suboptimal, then efforts should be made to identify the barriers to usage and alternative therapies may need to be considered. A repeat PSG may be indicated if symptoms persist or worsen with good adherence or there has been a significant change in weight or cardiopulmonary status.

The use of PAP has revolutionized the care of patients with sleep-disordered breathing. For OSAS, PAP clearly improves respiratory disturbances,[7] daytime sleepiness,[8,9] cognitive impairment,[10] mood,[11] and quality of life[12]; reduces automobile accidents[13,14]; and improves cardiovascular sequela, such as systemic hypertension.[15–17] Respiratory assist devices have advanced to the point that they can measure patients' respiratory parameters and can provide feedback in a closed-loop system to manipulate the output variables. Because the devices are complex, it is important for health care providers to have a working knowledge of the different modes and algorithms to optimize the care of each patient. Despite the proven efficacy of PAP therapy, patient adherence remains a challenge. Educational, supportive, and behavioral interventions along with the use of comfort features and minimizing of adverse side effects play an important role in improving adherence.

## REFERENCES

1. Sullivan CE, Issa FG, Berthon-Jones M, et al. Reversal of obstructive sleep apnoea by continuous positive airway pressure applied through the nares. Lancet 1981;1:862–5.

2. Strohl KP, Redline S. Nasal CPAP therapy, upper airway muscle activation, and obstructive sleep apnea. Am Rev Respir Dis 1986;134:555–8.

3. Van de Graaff WB. Thoracic influence on upper airway patency. J Appl Physiol (1985) 1988;65:2124–31.

4. Kushida CA, Littner MR, Hirshkowitz M, et al. Practice parameters for the use of continuous and bilevel positive airway pressure devices to treat adult patients with sleep-related breathing disorders. Sleep 2006;29:375–80.

5. Loube DI, Gay PC, Strohl KP, et al. Indications for positive airway pressure treatment of adult obstructive sleep apnea patients: a consensus statement. Chest 1999;115:863–6.

6. Epstein LJ, Kristo D, Strollo PJ Jr, et al. Clinical guideline for the evaluation, management and long-term care of obstructive sleep apnea in adults. J Clin Sleep Med 2009;5:263–76.

7. Loredo JS, Ancoli-Israel S, Dimsdale JE. Effect of continuous positive airway pressure vs placebo continuous positive airway pressure on sleep quality in obstructive sleep apnea. Chest 1999;116:1545–9.

8. Sforza E, Krieger J. Daytime sleepiness after long-term continuous positive airway pressure (CPAP) treatment in obstructive sleep apnea syndrome. J Neurol Sci 1992;110:21–6.

9. Chin K, Fukuhara S, Takahashi K, et al. Response shift in perception of sleepiness in obstructive sleep apnea-hypopnea syndrome before and after treatment with nasal CPAP. Sleep 2004;27:490–3.

10. Kushida CA, Nichols DA, Holmes TH, et al. Effects of continuous positive airway pressure on neurocognitive function in obstructive sleep apnea patients: the Apnea Positive Pressure Long-term Efficacy Study (APPLES). Sleep 2012;35:1593–602.

11. El-Sherbini AM, Bediwy AS, El-Mitwalli A. Association between obstructive sleep apnea (OSA) and depression and the effect of continuous positive airway pressure (CPAP) treatment. Neuropsychiatr Dis Treat 2011;7:715–21.

12. Barnes M, McEvoy RD, Banks S, et al. Efficacy of positive airway pressure and oral appliance in mild to moderate obstructive sleep apnea. Am J Respir Crit Care Med 2004;170:656–64.

13. Findley L, Smith C, Hooper J, et al. Treatment with nasal CPAP decreases automobile accidents in patients with sleep apnea. Am J Respir Crit Care Med 2000;161:857–9.

14. Antonopoulos CN, Sergentanis TN, Daskalopoulou SS, et al. Nasal continuous positive airway pressure (nCPAP) treatment for obstructive sleep apnea, road traffic accidents and driving simulator performance: a meta-analysis. Sleep Med Rev 2011;15:301–10.

15. Jaimchariyatam N, Rodriguez CL, Budur K. Does CPAP treatment in mild obstructive sleep apnea affect blood pressure? Sleep Med 2010;11:837–42.

16. Jennum P, Wildschiodtz G, Christensen NJ, et al. Blood pressure, catecholamines, and pancreatic polypeptide in obstructive sleep apnea with and without nasal Continuous Positive Airway Pressure (nCPAP) treatment. Am J Hypertens 1989;2:847–52.

17. Gay P, Weaver T, Loube D, et al. Evaluation of positive airway pressure treatment for sleep related breathing disorders in adults. Sleep 2006;29:381–401.

18. Chai CL, Pathinathan A, Smith B. Continuous positive airway pressure delivery interfaces for obstructive sleep apnoea. Cochrane Database Syst Rev 2006;(4):CD005308.

19. Massie CA, Hart RW. Clinical outcomes related to interface type in patients with obstructive sleep apnea/hypopnea syndrome who are using continuous positive airway pressure. Chest 2003;123:1112–8.

20. Anderson FE, Kingshott RN, Taylor DR, et al. A randomized crossover efficacy trial of oral CPAP (Oracle) compared with nasal CPAP in the management of obstructive sleep apnea. Sleep 2003;26:721–6.
21. Martins De Araujo MT, Vieira SB, Vasquez EC, et al. Heated humidification or face mask to prevent upper airway dryness during continuous positive airway pressure therapy. Chest 2000;117:142–7.
22. Kushida CA, Chediak A, Berry RB, et al. Clinical guidelines for the manual titration of positive airway pressure in patients with obstructive sleep apnea. J Clin Sleep Med 2008;4:157–71.
23. Piper AJ, Wang D, Yee BJ, et al. Randomised trial of CPAP vs bilevel support in the treatment of obesity hypoventilation syndrome without severe nocturnal desaturation. Thorax 2008;63:395–401.
24. Marcus CL, Rosen G, Ward SL, et al. Adherence to and effectiveness of positive airway pressure therapy in children with obstructive sleep apnea. Pediatrics 2006;117:e442–51.
25. Resta O, Guido P, Picca V, et al. Prescription of nCPAP and nBIPAP in obstructive sleep apnoea syndrome: Italian experience in 105 subjects. a prospective two centre study. Respir Med 1998;92:820–7.
26. Ballard RD, Gay PC, Strollo PJ. Interventions to improve compliance in sleep apnea patients previously non-compliant with continuous positive airway pressure. J Clin Sleep Med 2007;3:706–12.
27. Littner M, Hirshkowitz M, Davila D, et al. Practice parameters for the use of auto-titrating continuous positive airway pressure devices for titrating pressures and treating adult patients with obstructive sleep apnea syndrome. An American Academy of Sleep Medicine report. Sleep 2002;25:143–7.
28. Senn O, Brack T, Russi EW, et al. A continuous positive airway pressure trial as a novel approach to the diagnosis of the obstructive sleep apnea syndrome. Chest 2006;129:67–75.
29. Morgenthaler TI, Aurora RN, Brown T, et al. Practice parameters for the use of autotitrating continuous positive airway pressure devices for titrating pressures and treating adult patients with obstructive sleep apnea syndrome: an update for 2007. An American Academy of Sleep Medicine report. Sleep 2008;31:141–7.
30. Ip S, D'Ambrosio C, Patel K, et al. Auto-titrating versus fixed continuous positive airway pressure for the treatment of obstructive sleep apnea: a systematic review with meta-analyses. Syst Rev 2012;1:20.
31. Patruno V, Aiolfi S, Costantino G, et al. Fixed and autoadjusting continuous positive airway pressure treatments are not similar in reducing cardiovascular risk factors in patients with obstructive sleep apnea. Chest 2007;131:1393–9.
32. Patruno V, Tobaldini E, Bianchi AM, et al. Acute effects of autoadjusting and fixed continuous positive airway pressure treatments on cardiorespiratory coupling in obese patients with obstructive sleep apnea. Eur J Intern Med 2014;25:164–8.
33. Carlucci A, Ceriana P, Mancini M, et al. Efficacy of bilevel-auto treatment in patients with obstructive sleep apnea not responsive to or intolerant of continuous positive airway pressure ventilation. J Clin Sleep Med 2015;11(9):981–5.
34. Aloia MS, Stanchina M, Arnedt JT, et al. Treatment adherence and outcomes in flexible vs standard continuous positive airway pressure therapy. Chest 2005;127:2085–93.
35. Bakker JP, Marshall NS. Flexible pressure delivery modification of continuous positive airway pressure for obstructive sleep apnea does not improve compliance with therapy: systematic review and meta-analysis. Chest 2011;139:1322–30.

36. Chihara Y, Tsuboi T, Hitomi T, et al. Flexible positive airway pressure improves treatment adherence compared with auto-adjusting PAP. Sleep 2013;36:229–36.

37. Murphy PB, Davidson C, Hind MD, et al. Volume targeted versus pressure support non-invasive ventilation in patients with super obesity and chronic respiratory failure: a randomised controlled trial. Thorax 2012;67:727–34.

38. Galetke W, Ghassemi BM, Priegnitz C, et al. Anticyclic modulated ventilation versus continuous positive airway pressure in patients with coexisting obstructive sleep apnea and Cheyne-Stokes respiration: a randomized crossover trial. Sleep Med 2014;15:874–9.

39. Randerath WJ, Javaheri S. Adaptive servoventilation in central sleep apnea. Sleep Med Clin 2014;9:69–85.

40. Medicine AAoS. Special safety notice: ASV therapy for central sleep apnea patients with heart failure. Available at: http://aasmnet.org/articles.aspx?id=5562.

41. Kalan A, Kenyon GS, Seemungal TA, et al. Adverse effects of nasal continuous positive airway pressure therapy in sleep apnoea syndrome. J Laryngol Otol 1999;113:888–92.

42. Pepin JL, Leger P, Veale D, et al. Side effects of nasal continuous positive airway pressure in sleep apnea syndrome. Study of 193 patients in two French sleep centers. Chest 1995;107:375–81.

43. Jarjour NN, Wilson P. Pneumocephalus associated with nasal continuous positive airway pressure in a patient with sleep apnea syndrome. Chest 1989;96:1425–6.

44. Strollo PJ Jr, Sanders MH, Atwood CW. Positive pressure therapy. Clin Chest Med 1998;19:55–68.

45. Lehman S, Antic NA, Thompson C, et al. Central sleep apnea on commencement of continuous positive airway pressure in patients with a primary diagnosis of obstructive sleep apnea-hypopnea. J Clin Sleep Med 2007;3:462–6.

46. Javaheri S, Smith J, Chung E. The prevalence and natural history of complex sleep apnea. J Clin Sleep Med 2009;5:205–11.

47. Morgenthaler TI, Kuzniar TJ, Wolfe LF, et al. The complex sleep apnea resolution study: a prospective randomized controlled trial of continuous positive airway pressure versus adaptive servoventilation therapy. Sleep 2014;37:927–34.

48. Furukawa T, Suzuki M, Ochiai M, et al. Long-term adherence to nasal continuous positive airway pressure therapy by hypertensive patients with preexisting sleep apnea. J Cardiol 2014;63:281–5.

49. O'Donnell AR, Bjornson CL, Bohn SG, et al. Compliance rates in children using noninvasive continuous positive airway pressure. Sleep 2006;29:651–8.

50. Weaver TE, Grunstein RR. Adherence to continuous positive airway pressure therapy: the challenge to effective treatment. Proc Am Thorac Soc 2008;5:173–8.

51. Kribbs NB, Pack AI, Kline LR, et al. Objective measurement of patterns of nasal CPAP use by patients with obstructive sleep apnea. Am Rev Respir Dis 1993;147: 887–95.

52. Stepnowsky CJ Jr, Moore PJ. Nasal CPAP treatment for obstructive sleep apnea: developing a new perspective on dosing strategies and compliance. J Psychosom Res 2003;54:599–605.

53. National Coverage Determination (NCD) for Continuous Positive Airway Pressure (CPAP) Therapy For Obstructive Sleep Apnea (OSA) 3/13/2008. 2015. Available at: www.cms.gov.

54. Weaver TE, Kribbs NB, Pack AI, et al. Night-to-night variability in CPAP use over the first three months of treatment. Sleep 1997;20:278–83.

55. Neill AM, Wai HS, Bannan SP, et al. Humidified nasal continuous positive airway pressure in obstructive sleep apnoea. Eur Respir J 2003;22:258–62.

56. Massie CA, Hart RW, Peralez K, et al. Effects of humidification on nasal symptoms and compliance in sleep apnea patients using continuous positive airway pressure. Chest 1999;116:403–8.
57. Wozniak DR, Lasserson TJ, Smith I. Educational, supportive and behavioural interventions to improve usage of continuous positive airway pressure machines in adults with obstructive sleep apnoea. Cochrane Database Syst Rev 2014;(1):CD007736.
58. Lai AY, Fong DY, Lam JC, et al. The efficacy of a brief motivational enhancement education program on CPAP adherence in OSA: a randomized controlled trial. Chest 2014;146:600–10.
59. Olsen S, Smith S, Oei TP. Adherence to continuous positive airway pressure therapy in obstructive sleep apnoea sufferers: a theoretical approach to treatment adherence and intervention. Clin Psychol Rev 2008;28:1355–71.
60. Koontz KL, Slifer KJ, Cataldo MD, et al. Improving pediatric compliance with positive airway pressure therapy: the impact of behavioral intervention. Sleep 2003;26:1010–5.
61. Hoy CJ, Vennelle M, Kingshott RN, et al. Can intensive support improve continuous positive airway pressure use in patients with the sleep apnea/hypopnea syndrome? Am J Respir Crit Care Med 1999;159:1096–100.
62. Hui DS, Choy DK, Li TS, et al. Determinants of continuous positive airway pressure compliance in a group of Chinese patients with obstructive sleep apnea. Chest 2001;120:170–6.

# Oral Appliances in Obstructive Sleep Apnea

Anthony Dioguardi, DMD[a],*, Moh'd Al-Halawani, MD[b]

## KEYWORDS

- Obstructive sleep apnea • Snoring • Oral appliance therapy
- Mandibular advancement device • Temporomandibular joint • Home sleep testing
- Bruxism • Dental sleep medicine

## KEY POINTS

- Oral appliance therapy (OAT) should be considered for appropriate patients who request treatment of primary snoring or obstructive sleep apnea and express a preference for OAT rather than alternative treatment.
- Patients who are considered appropriate for OAT should ideally have a minimum of 10 healthy, well-supported and distributed teeth of sufficient size and contour in each arch; and have a stable temporomandibular joint system without pain or restriction during lateral or protrusive excursions.
- Dentists who treat patients with sleep disorders require advanced training in dental sleep medicine, which is not commonly provided in dental school or residency programs.
- There are many types of oral appliances available, and these should be selected from patient anatomy, physiology, sleep behavior, and preferences.
- Patients who have been treated with OAT should maintain long-term follow-up care with both dentists and physicians beyond the initial adjustment period.

## BACKGROUND

Oral appliances for the treatment of airway obstruction were first addressed in 1923 in the literature by French pediatrician, Pierre Robin,[1] who described the fall of the base of the tongue as the cause of nasopharyngeal impairment and proposed a prosthetic device to correct "the dysmorphic atresia of the mandible." However, these appliances were not commonly used for the treatment of sleep disordered breathing until the early 1980s, when a tongue-retaining device for the treatment of snoring and sleep

Conflicts of Interest: The authors have no commercial conflicts of interest.
[a] Sleep Apnea and Snoring Dental Therapy of Connecticut, 123 York Street, Suite 2J, New Haven, CT 06511, USA; [b] Sleep Medicine Fellowship Program, Section of Pulmonary, Critical Care and Sleep Medicine, Yale University School of Medicine, 20 York Street, New Haven, CT 06510, USA
* Corresponding author.
E-mail address: adioguardi01@gmail.com

apnea was described by Cartwright and Samelson.[2] This device was followed by renewed interest in mandibular advancement devices (MADs) that reposition the mandible in a protrusive position in order to help maintain the patency of the upper airway during sleep.

The ensuing popular demand for these appliances led to a plethora of appliance designs being targeted to both the dental professional and directly to the general population seeking relief from snoring. The US Food and Drug Administration (FDA) has classified over-the-counter antisnoring mouth guards as class II medical devices, which places restrictions on their sale without prescription by a physician. Although this classification was challenged and upheld in *United States v Snoring Relief Labs Of America* (manufacturer of SnorBan an OTC mouthpiece), these devices continue to be readily available over the Internet, taking advantage of the FDA exemptions from adequate directions for use, which require consumers to appropriately answer a questionnaire before fulfilling an order. The variety of available devices also led to much confusion among practitioners and third-party payers as to which features of appliances were fundamental to treatment success.[3]

In 2014, the American Academy of Dental Sleep Medicine (AADSM) released a position paper designed to address these issues and define the characteristics of an effective MAD.[4]

### Mechanism of Oral Appliance Therapy Action

A mandibular advancement device functions by protruding and stabilizing the mandible in order to maintain a patent upper airway during sleep.[4] The precise physiologic and anatomic changes that result from mandibular advancement remain elusive.

Tsuiki and colleagues[5] reported that the protruded mandible results in changes in the anteroposterior width of the upper airway, and positions of the hyoid bone and the third cervical vertebra. However, Ryan and colleagues[6] reported that MAD use resulted in an increase in the lateral dimension of the velopharynx greater than the increase in the anteroposterior dimension (**Fig. 1**).

Various clinical attributes have been associated with successful treatment outcome. These attributes include younger age, female sex, less severe obstructive sleep apnea (OSA), supine-dependent OSA, lower body mass index, and smaller neck circumference.[7,8]

Analysis of lateral cephalometric images have shown an association between certain characteristics, such as retrognathic mandible, lower hyoid position, and greater angle between the cranial base and mandibular plane, with favorable MAD outcomes. However, none of the cephalometric associations are considered strong enough to have any clinically significant predictive value.[9]

In short, there is currently no reliable way to predict who will respond positively to MAD based on observable clinical features. In some patients, mandibular advancement results in improvement in the airway obstruction, whereas in others it results in increased obstruction.[10] However, Remmers and colleagues[11] reported predicting MAD therapeutic success using a remotely controlled mandibular positioning device during polysomnography.

### Definition of an Effective Oral Appliance

The abundance of trademarked custom MAD appliances available on the market all share the common characteristic of protrusively repositioning the mandible. Differences in materials, weight, size, range, placement of protrusive element, and a host

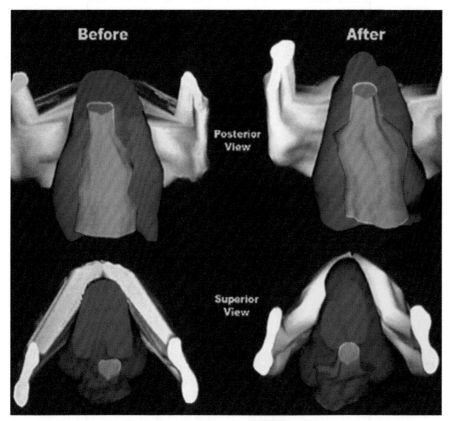

**Fig. 1.** Three-dimensional reconstruction of the velopharynx before and after MAD use. Red: tongue; white: mandible; blue: airway. (*Courtesy of* Alan A. Lowe, DMD, PhD, FRCD, Vancouver, British Columbia.)

of other factors provide dentists with a wide variety of appliance choices to accommodate patients' physiologies and preferences (**Table 1**). Studies support that custom-made, adjustable MADs are superior in efficacy to prefabricated and nonadjustable alternatives.[12,13] The tongue-retaining device has similar efficacy but lower compliance than the MAD, but remains an option for significantly or partially edentulous patients.[14]

In 2014, the AADSM published a position report defining what constituted an effective oral appliance for the treatment of OSA in an effort set the standard of care and provide scientific rationale for the inclusion or exclusion of various device parameters.[4]

This article defined an effective oral appliance as one that:

- Has a dual arch design
- Is adjustable in a way that permits gradual protrusive advancement over a range of at least 5 mm
- Has an expected lifespan of at least 3 years
- Has a mechanism of protrusion that is verifiable and reversible
- Is custom fabricated for optimum fit and comfort

**Table 1**
The variations of some commonly used MAD designs

| | | | | |
|---|---|---|---|---|
| Materials | Laser-sintered polyamide 12 body, polyamide 11 removable bars | Acrylic resin, stainless steel screw mechanism and bar | Acrylic resin, stainless steel screw mechanism | Control cured Poly (methyl methacrylate) |
| Protrusive mechanism | Replaceable bars of marked length | Telescopic fixed bar, adjustment screw on upper element with millimeter ruler | Fixed dorsal fin, adjustment screw on lower element | Fixed dorsal fin, no moving parts |
| Protrusive range | 15 mm in 0.5-mm increments | 8 mm, continuously variable | 5 mm, continuously variable | 2 upper and 2 lower interchangeable elements for a maximum of 3 different positions |

## Efficacy

Several studies provide evidence for the efficacy of MADs in reducing the overall apnea-hypopnea index [AHI], but with lower effectiveness compared with continuous positive airway pressure (CPAP). Treatment success across all levels of OSA severity using MADs is around 50%, with an overall average reduction in baseline AHI of 55%. MADs were also shown to have a positive effect on snoring and daytime symptoms, decreasing excessive daytime sleepiness and improving quality of life compared with placebo.[8,12,13,15] These results were more evident when the MADs were custom made compared with prefabricated ones.[16]

In a recent meta-analysis, Sutherland and colleagues[17] showed that 37% of patients using MADs achieved an AHI less than 5/h, 52% achieved AHI less than 10/h, and 64% reduced AHI by greater than or equal to 50%. Response rates were lower in patients with severe OSA; however, 70% of those showed a reduction in AHI greater than or equal to 50%, and 23% had complete resolution of OSA.

## Compliance

MADs have higher compliance rates than CPAP with a median use of 77% of nights during the first year.[15,18] A short-term study by Philips and colleagues[18] showed that subjective reports of nightly compliance were less for CPAP compared with MAD.

## Side Effects of Mandibular Advancement Devices

MAD use is usually associated with mild and transient side effects that tend to resolve within several days or weeks, given that the device has a good fit and is used by the patient regularly.[19]

Commonly reported side effects include:

- Temporomandibular joint (TMJ) discomfort or pain
- Myofascial pain
- Tooth tenderness
- Excessive salivation
- Gum irritation and bleeding
- Dry mouth

Occasionally, side effects negatively affect treatment compliance, but significant and persistent side effects are rare.[13,15]

Long-term MAD use may lead to dental and skeletal side effects that include:

- Decrease in overjet and overbite
- Retroclination of the maxillary incisors
- Proclination of the mandibular incisors
- Increases in the mandibular plane angle
- Increases in the anterior facial height
- Decrease in the number of occlusal contact points
- Anteroposterior change in occlusion[20,21]

Morning jaw exercises following MAD use have been shown to:

- Improve compliance
- Reduce side effects
- Improve quality of life
- Reduce sleep symptoms
- Alleviate muscle stiffness
- Aid in the mandible returning to its normal position[22,23]

## Hybrid Therapy

The use of a hybrid therapy combining nasal CPAP with MAD therapy for patients with OSA has been reported in the literature. Thornton[24] reported the first case in 2002 of combined MAD and CPAP therapy in a patient with severe OSA who initially could not tolerate treatment with CPAP because of increased pressures and leakage, and later failed treatment with MAD because of TMJ symptoms at maximum protrusion. The combination therapy was better tolerated by the patient with fewer side effects, because the combination therapy allowed for the use of a lower CPAP pressure and less advancement of the MAD.

This treatment strategy leads to reduced CPAP pressure, better fit, less leakage, and greater compliance.[24]

Another case report was published by Denbar[25]; both reports agree that MADs increase the upper airway size, decreasing the need for high CPAP pressures to maintain airway patency with combination therapy, and leading to better tolerance than with CPAP or MAD alone.

A study by El-Solh and colleagues[26] in 2010 included 10 patients who were using MAD therapy for OSA after they could not tolerate CPAP and still had incomplete response to treatment. This study showed that combination therapy was well tolerated by all patients and resulted in a reduction of CPAP pressure and AHI by 29% and 86% respectively from baseline.[26]

This finding suggests that combination therapy may be effective in patients who cannot tolerate treatment with either CPAP or MAD alone.

## Patient Selection

### Clinical examination of oral appliance candidates

An oral examination preceding a referral to a dentist for oral appliance therapy (OAT) should include evaluation of the overall condition of the existing dentition, their supporting structures, the TMJ, and health of the soft tissue (**Box 1**).

### Dental Caries and Oral Appliance Therapy

The teeth that support an MAD should be free from active dental caries, periodontally healthy, and structurally sound in order to withstand the forces resisting the displacement of the arch over the long term.[27–29]

Evaluation of potential MAD candidates should include a complete intraoral examination that includes visual inspection of the teeth for caries, structural compromise, and their supporting tissues. Advanced dental decay can result in the devitalization of the pulp chamber, which can in turn lead to pain that is exacerbated by tapping

---

**Box 1**
**Characteristics of an ideal oral appliance candidate**

- No active dental decay or periodontitis.
- A stable dentition with at least 10 well-supported teeth well distributed in each arch.
- A healthy TMJ complex with pain-free and unrestricted protrusive, lateral, and vertical excursive movements.
- Has been diagnosed with OSA and expresses a desire for a nonsurgical alternative to positive airway pressure treatment.
- Expresses a desire for a nonsurgical treatment of primary snoring.

the affected tooth with a mirror handle or similar instrument. These necrotic chambers often drain to the buccal and lingual surfaces, resulting in a draining fistula adjacent to the affected root (**Fig. 2**).[30]

The use of a removable oral appliance can lead to increased tooth decay by acting as a new retentive surface for the colonization of *Streptococcus mutans* and other cariogenic bacteria.[31] In addition, any appliance that covers the surface of the teeth has the potential to compromise the caries-protective cleansing effect of saliva, which can lead to an increased rate of dental caries.[32] Likewise, xerostomia (dry mouth), immune suppression, or any other condition that reduces the ability to resist dental decay or periodontal inflammation should be addressed before referral for an oral appliance.[33,34]

### Can the Existing Teeth Support a Dental Appliance?

MADs reposition the mandibular arch to a protrusive position, and place a protrusive force on the lower teeth and an equal and opposite retrusive force on the upper teeth. In addition, oral appliances that have the upper element connected to the lower element by a hinge, bar, or elastic can act to dislodge the appliance when the mouth is opened. Accordingly, the teeth retaining the appliance should be large enough, adequately secured in bone, and possess the physical undercuts necessary to resist the various forces placed on the appliance.

Although a minimum of 10 healthy teeth per arch is traditionally considered the general requirement to retain most types of tooth-borne MADs, it must be considered that not all teeth provide equal resistance to unwanted tooth movement, also known as anchorage.[35] This anchorage is generally related to the size and root area of the teeth that are secured to bone, with the canines and molars providing significantly greater anchorage than the smaller rooted incisors and bicuspids.[36]

In situations in which natural undercuts are inadequate to retain an MAD, dentists can alter the contour of the teeth either by enameloplasty or the addition of composite resin (**Fig. 3**), creating undercuts that enable satisfactory retention of the appliance. In addition, if teeth are not well distributed throughout the arch, the resulting forces will be disproportionality distributed as well.

Anchorage can be compromised by periodontitis or occlusal trauma, which can lead to the loss of the tooth's bony support (**Fig. 4**). The root of a tooth is anchored to the supporting bone by a periodontal ligament, which is attached to both the tooth

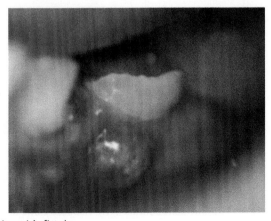

**Fig. 2.** Dental caries with fistula.

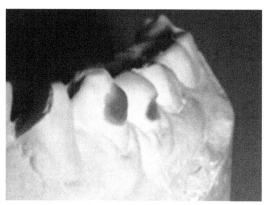

**Fig. 3.** Short teeth and bonded undercuts; enameloplasty shown in pink and addition of composite resin in blue.

and supporting bone. In many cases, a tooth becomes visibly mobile because of secondary occlusal forces overcoming the ability of the tooth to resist those forces.[37] Exceptions to the paradigm that only teeth can retain an MAD are discussed in reports of MAD designs that secure their retention by means of dental implants, extraoral soft tissue, and the edentulous arch.[38–40]

Periodontitis can often appear as red, swollen gingiva adjacent to the teeth, and readily bleeds on probing. In other cases, the disease exists without signs of obvious surface inflammation, with the inflammatory process existing beneath the surface of the gingiva in the space adjacent to the tooth, known as the periodontal pocket (**Fig. 5**). Tooth mobility can easily be observed by applying gentle pressure with a mirror handle. Active periodontitis and/or mobility in 1 or more of the teeth can be

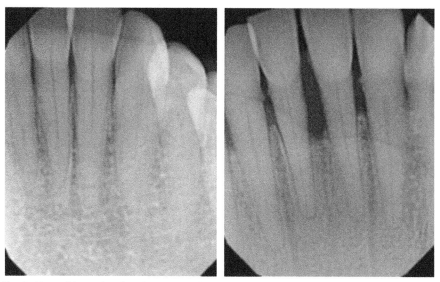

**Fig. 4.** Normal bone level without periodontitis (*left*). Reduced bone level and anchorage secondary to periodontitis (*right*).

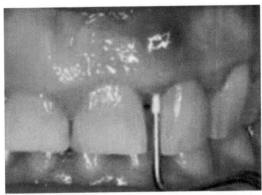

**Fig. 5.** Periodontal probe revealing loss of bone mesial of tooth 9. Note draining fistula buccal to base of the periodontal pocket.

exacerbated by the use of an oral appliance and must be addressed before fabrication of the device is considered. Clearly, patients presenting with a high caries rate and/or active periodontal disease, coupled with a history of only emergency-related dental visits, are better served by alternative therapies for their sleep disordered breathing.

### Bruxism and Oral Appliance Therapy

The presence of teeth with flattened occlusal surfaces suggests a history of or active tooth grinding or bruxism, a condition that has been associated with sleep apnea.[41] The precise nature of this association, or whether or not there is a causal relationship between bruxism and OSA, remains unclear.[42] Bruxism (**Fig. 6**) is commonly evaluated during polysomnography by electrodes placed on the masseter muscle, but is not typically evaluated during type 3 home sleep testing.[43,44] Nocturnal bruxism commonly results in breakage of acrylic oral appliances (**Fig. 7**) and its presence suggests that the device should be fabricated from one of the newer, more durable materials.[45]

### Temporomandibular Joint Considerations in Oral Appliance Therapy

A healthy TMJ complex that enables the patient to have pain-free and unrestricted protrusive, lateral, and vertical movement is a prerequisite for any OAT. It is

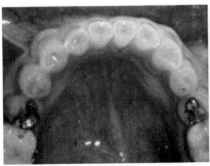
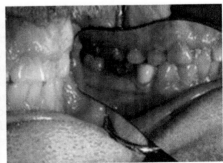

**Fig. 6.** Bruxism; note the characteristic wear pattern on the lower incisors (*left*); and loss of vertical dimension resulting from destruction of the incisal portion of the dentition (*right*).

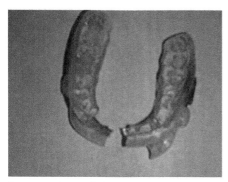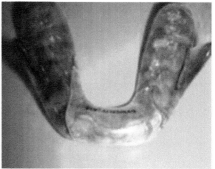

**Fig. 7.** Appliance failure secondary to nocturnal bruxism.

unreasonable to expect a patient to wear an MAD if it is uncomfortable. Therefore, careful consideration must be given before attempting fabrication of an MAD for a patient with significant pain or restrictions when entering protrusive, lateral, or vertical mandibular excursions. Clinical evaluation of the TMJ complex should include observation of anything suggestive of disorder during these excursions (clicks, pops, or pain). In addition, the muscles of mastication, including the temporalis, masseter, and internal pterygoid, should be palpated and any tenderness noted.[46]

### Which Patients with Sleep Disorder Should Be Referred for Oral Appliance Therapy?

The July 2015 American Academy of Sleep Medicine (AASM)/AADSM guidelines[47] recommend that oral appliances should be offered to adult patients:

- Who request treatment of primary snoring (without sleep apnea)
  - The guideline recommends that patients who have failed traditional conservative measures such as positional therapy, weight loss, and alcohol avoidance be offered OAT.
  - Because loud snoring is often a warning sign of underlying OSA,[48] the diagnosis of primary snoring should be made by a sleep physician rather than a dentist. This notion has recently been challenged by the Texas Board of Dental Examiners, which passed Rule 108.12 referring to sleep studies as a screening tool that dentists may use to differentiate OSA from primary snoring and left it to the dentists' discretion to determine which patients require physician assessment before the initiation of treatment. In response, the Texas Medical Association and the AASM are currently challenging the ruling and requested the court to void the rule. This challenge has been supported by the AADSM, which maintains that treatment by a dentist may proceed only after a diagnosis of OSA or snoring has been made by a physician.[28]
- Are intolerant or prefer an alternative treatment to CPAP therapy
  - This new guideline no longer differentiates between different levels of OSA (mild, moderate, and severe). This recommendation was based on a meta-analysis of past studies that showed no statistically significant difference in the mean reduction in AHI before and after treatment in patients using oral appliances versus CPAP across all levels of OSA severity. However, the probability of achieving a target AHI in patients with moderate to severe OSA is significantly greater with CPAP than OAT.[47]

### Treatment Protocol and the Dental Referral

OAT should be undertaken by a qualified dentist only after a referral from a qualified physician trained in sleep medicine who has performed a face-to-face evaluation of the patient.[49]

Dentists who treat patients with sleep disorders require advanced training in dental sleep medicine, which is not commonly provided in dental school or residency programs. The AASM/AADSM defines a qualified dentist as one who has completed 25 hours of continuing education in dental sleep medicine within the past 2 years from a nonprofit organization, been designated a dental director of an accredited dental sleep medicine facility by a nonprofit organization, or has certification in dental sleep medicine from a nonprofit organization.[47]

The dental evaluation for OAT should include examination of the oral cavity including the teeth and their supporting structures, soft tissue, temporomandibular complex, and review of a recent complete dental radiographic survey. A medical and sleep history should be taken and sleep studies reviewed. A thorough review of informed consent that includes the benefits, alternatives, potential side effects, and risks of the proposed therapy, along with the risks inherent in not treating the condition, should be reviewed in detail and signed by the patient in the presence of a witness.

Various options in appliances should be discussed, as should the dentist's recommendation of the appliance that would be ideally suited for that patient based on the clinical examination and the patient's preferences. It is highly advantageous for the patient to have the opportunity to physically hold and examine demonstration models of the appliances. Although CPAP has been consistently proved to be more predictably effective in treating moderate to severe OSA than OAT,[50] it must be remembered that the primary reason most patients seek out OAT is because they expect to be able to tolerate it better than they would a CPAP device. It is intuitively obvious that patients are even more likely to be compliant with a device that they have had a part in choosing.

The postinsertion adjustment period typically involves at least several visits over approximately 3 months before referral back to the sleep physician to confirm efficacy. During this time, the protrusive settings are gradually increased to what the dentist determines (by both subjective and sometimes objective means) to be the ideal therapeutic position.

The current clinical guidelines stress open communication between dentist and physician, OAT efficacy confirmation by physician-ordered sleep testing, and short-term and long-term medical and dental follow-up once efficacy has been established. Once the physician has verified that the OAT is effectively treating the patient's condition, the AADSM recommends that patients be seen a minimum of once every 6 months for the first 2 years and then on a once-a-year basis.[51] During these visits, the dentist can:

- Monitor the physical integrity of the appliance
- Reassess the patient's subjective symptoms, such as snoring and sleepiness as measured by the Epworth Sleepiness Scale
- Evaluate potential side effects of the device, such as bite changes (by comparing with preliminary models, radiographs and photographs), caries, and temporomandibular dysfunction
- Refer the patient back to the sleep physician if there are reasons to think that the current treatment is no longer effective

## Home Sleep Testing in the Dental Setting

The AADSM Protocol for Oral Appliance Therapy for Sleep Disordered Breathing in Adults: An Update for 2012,[52] states that, "After this initial fitting, the dentist may obtain objective data during an initial trial period using a portable monitor to verify that the oral appliance effectively improves upper airway patency during sleep by enlarging the upper airway and/or decreasing upper airway collapsibility. If necessary, the dentist makes further adjustments to the device during a final fitting to ensure that optimal fit and positioning have been attained."

Type 3 or type 4 home sleep tests (HSTs) are commonly given to patients by qualified dentists seeking to adjust the appliances to achieve the optimal desired effect of upper airway patency. Various protrusive and vertical positions can be assessed in order to adjust the appliance to result in optimal sleep scores. This objective information becomes particularly useful in cases in which the patient does not experience subjective symptoms such as snoring or daytime sleepiness. These tests are commonly scored by computer algorithm, and although not diagnostic, can provide valuable comparative information with respect to appliance settings.

It must be stressed to the patient that dentist-administered HSTs are performed solely to aid the dentist in the adjustment of the appliance and are not diagnostic, because the diagnosis of medical conditions is not within the ethical or legal scope of the practice of dentistry. It is the opinion of this author that, before a dentist gives an HST to a patient, the patient must agree in writing that the patient understands that the results of the test will not be shared directly with the patient, but may be shared with the patient's sleep physician.

## SUMMARY

OAT use has become an increasingly popular option in the treatment of primary snoring and OSA in recent years. Although less consistently effective than CPAP, it remains an attractive nonsurgical treatment option because of its high levels of compliance, convenience, and stealth. A focused oral examination can help determine whether or not a patient is a candidate for an MAD. Recent studies have suggested that CPAP and OAT used together can provide a higher level of success than either used alone.

## REFERENCES

1. Robin P. A fall of the base of the tongue considered as a new cause of nasopharyngeal respiratory impairment: Pierre Robin sequence, a translation. 1923. Plast Reconstr Surg 1994;93(6):1301–3.
2. Cartwright RD, Samelson CF. The effects of a nonsurgical treatment for obstructive sleep apnea. The tongue-retaining device. JAMA 1982;248(6):705–9.
3. Food and Drug Administration. Food and Drug Administration, Department of Health and Human Services. Code of Federal Regulations Title 21, Sec. 801.109 Prescription devices. 2015. Available at: http://www.accessdata.fda.gov/scripts/cdrh/cfdocs/cfcfr/cfrsearch.cfm?fr=801.109. Accessed March 13, 2016.
4. Scherr SC, Dort LC, Almeida FR, et al. Definition of an effective oral appliance for the treatment of obstructive sleep apnea and snoring: a report of the American Academy of Dental Sleep Medicine. J Dent Sleep Med 2014;1(1):51.
5. Tsuiki S, Hiyama S, Ono T, et al. Effects of a titratable oral appliance on supine airway size in awake non-apneic individuals. Sleep 2001;24(5):554–60.

6. Ryan CF, Love LL, Peat D, et al. Mandibular advancement oral appliance therapy for obstructive sleep apnoea: effect on awake calibre of the velopharynx. Thorax 1999;54(11):972–7.

7. Blanco J, Zamarron C, Abeleira Pazos MT, et al. Prospective evaluation of an oral appliance in the treatment of obstructive sleep apnea syndrome. Sleep Breath 2005;9(1):20–5.

8. Marklund M, Stenlund H, Franklin KA. Mandibular advancement devices in 630 men and women with obstructive sleep apnea and snoring: tolerability and predictors of treatment success. Chest 2004;125(4):1270–8.

9. Ng AT, Darendeliler MA, Petocz P, et al. Cephalometry and prediction of oral appliance treatment outcome. Sleep Breath 2012;16(1):47–58.

10. Ferguson KA, Ono T, Lowe AA, et al. A short-term controlled trial of an adjustable oral appliance for the treatment of mild to moderate obstructive sleep apnoea. Thorax 1997;52(4):362–8.

11. Remmers J, Charkhandeh S, Grosse J, et al. Remotely controlled mandibular protrusion during sleep predicts therapeutic success with oral appliances in patients with obstructive sleep apnea. Sleep 2013;36(10):1517–25, 1525A.

12. Ahrens A, McGrath C, Hagg U. Subjective efficacy of oral appliance design features in the management of obstructive sleep apnea: a systematic review. Am J Orthod Dentofacial Orthop 2010;138(5):559–76.

13. Marklund M, Verbraecken J, Randerath W. Non-CPAP therapies in obstructive sleep apnoea: mandibular advancement device therapy. Eur Respir J 2012; 39(5):1241–7.

14. Deane SA, Cistulli PA, Ng AT, et al. Comparison of mandibular advancement splint and tongue stabilizing device in obstructive sleep apnea: a randomized controlled trial. Sleep 2009;32(5):648–53.

15. Ferguson KA, Cartwright R, Rogers R, et al. Oral appliances for snoring and obstructive sleep apnea: a review. Sleep 2006;29(2):244–62.

16. Serra-Torres S, Bellot-Arcis C, Montiel-Company JM, et al. Effectiveness of mandibular advancement appliances in treating obstructive sleep apnea syndrome: a systematic review. Laryngoscope 2016;126(2):507–14.

17. Sutherland K, Takaya H, Qian J, et al. Oral appliance treatment response and polysomnographic phenotypes of obstructive sleep apnea. J Clin Sleep Med 2015; 11(8):861–8.

18. Phillips CL, Grunstein RR, Darendeliler MA, et al. Health outcomes of continuous positive airway pressure versus oral appliance treatment for obstructive sleep apnea: a randomized controlled trial. Am J Respir Crit Care Med 2013;187(8): 879–87.

19. Aarab G, Lobbezoo F, Hamburger HL, et al. Effects of an oral appliance with different mandibular protrusion positions at a constant vertical dimension on obstructive sleep apnea. Clin Oral Investig 2010;14(3):339–45.

20. Doff MH, Finnema KJ, Hoekema A, et al. Long-term oral appliance therapy in obstructive sleep apnea syndrome: a controlled study on dental side effects. Clin Oral Investig 2013;17(2):475–82.

21. Wang X, Gong X, Yu Z, et al. Follow-up study of dental and skeletal changes in patients with obstructive sleep apnea and hypopnea syndrome with long-term treatment with the Silensor appliance. Am J Orthod Dentofacial Orthop 2015; 147(5):559–65.

22. Cunali PA, Almeida FR, Santos CD, et al. Mandibular exercises improve mandibular advancement device therapy for obstructive sleep apnea. Sleep Breath 2011;15(4):717–27.

23. Ueda H, Almeida FR, Chen H, et al. Effect of 2 jaw exercises on occlusal function in patients with obstructive sleep apnea during oral appliance therapy: a randomized controlled trial. Am J Orthod Dentofacial Orthop 2009;135(4):430.e1-7 [discussion: 430–1].

24. Thornton WK. Combined CPAP-oral appliance therapy: a case report. Sleep Review 2002. Available at: http://www.sleepreviewmag.com/2002/01/news-story-29/. Accessed August 6, 2016.

25. Denbar MA. A case study involving the combination treatment of an oral appliance and auto-titrating CPAP unit. Sleep Breath 2002;6(3):125–8.

26. El-Solh AA, Moitheennazima B, Akinnusi ME, et al. Combined oral appliance and positive airway pressure therapy for obstructive sleep apnea: a pilot study. Sleep Breath 2011;15(2):203–8.

27. Zlataric DK, Celebic A, Valentic-Peruzovic M. The effect of removable partial dentures on periodontal health of abutment and non-abutment teeth. J Periodontol 2002;73(2):137–44.

28. American Academy of Dental Sleep Medicine. President's message: dentistry's role in treating snoring and sleep apnea. 2014. Available at: http://www.aadsm.org/articles.aspx?id=5224. Accessed March 13, 2016.

29. Petit FX, Pepin JL, Bettega G, et al. Mandibular advancement devices: rate of contraindications in 100 consecutive obstructive sleep apnea patients. Am J Respir Crit Care Med 2002;166(3):274–8.

30. Johnson BR, Remeikis NA, Van Cura JE. Diagnosis and treatment of cutaneous facial sinus tracts of dental origin. J Am Dent Assoc 1999;130(6):832–6.

31. Batoni G, Pardini M, Giannotti A, et al. Effect of removable orthodontic appliances on oral colonisation by mutans streptococci in children. Eur J Oral Sci 2001;109(6):388–92.

32. Dowd FJ. Saliva and dental caries. Dent Clin North Am 1999;43(4):579–97.

33. Dreizen S, Brown LR, Daly TE, et al. Prevention of xerostomia-related dental caries in irradiated cancer patients. J Dent Res 1977;56(2):99–104.

34. Stanford TW, Rees TD. Acquired immune suppression and other risk factors/indicators for periodontal disease progression. Periodontol 2000 2003;32:118–35.

35. Kushida CA, Morgenthaler TI, Littner MR, et al. Practice parameters for the treatment of snoring and obstructive sleep apnea with oral appliances: an update for 2005. Sleep 2006;29(2):240–3.

36. Roberts-Harry D, Sandy J. Orthodontics. Part 9: anchorage control and distal movement. Br Dent J 2004;196(5):255–63.

37. Williams RC. Periodontal disease. N Engl J Med 1990;322(6):373–82.

38. Tripathi A, Gupta A, Tripathi S, et al. A novel use of complete denture prosthesis as mandibular advancement device in the treatment of obstructive sleep apnea in edentulous subjects. J Dent Sleep Med 2014;1(3):115–9.

39. Guimaraes TM, Colen S, Cunali PA, et al. Treatment of obstructive sleep apnea with mandibular advancement appliance over prostheses: a case report. Sleep Sci 2015;8(2):103–6.

40. Hoekema A, de Vries F, Heydenrijk K, et al. Implant-retained oral appliances: a novel treatment for edentulous patients with obstructive sleep apnea-hypopnea syndrome. Clin Oral Implants Res 2007;18(3):383–7.

41. Knight DJ, Leroux BG, Zhu C, et al. A longitudinal study of tooth wear in orthodontically treated patients. Am J Orthod Dentofacial Orthop 1997;112(2):194–202.

42. Balasubramaniam R, Klasser GD, Cistulli PA, et al. The link between sleep bruxism, sleep disordered breathing and temporomandibular disorders: an evidence-based review. J Dent Sleep Med 2014;1(1):27–37.

43. Saito M, Yamaguchi T, Mikami S, et al. Temporal association between sleep apnea–hypopnea and sleep bruxism events. J Sleep Res 2014;23:196–203. http://dx.doi.org/10.1111/jsr.12099.

44. Collop NA, Anderson WM, Boehlecke B, et al. Clinical guidelines for the use of unattended portable monitors in the diagnosis of obstructive sleep apnea in adult patients. Portable Monitoring Task Force of the American Academy of Sleep Medicine. J Clin Sleep Med 2007;3(7):737–47.

45. Landry-Schonbeck A, de Grandmont P, Rompre PH, et al. Effect of an adjustable mandibular advancement appliance on sleep bruxism: a crossover sleep laboratory study. Int J Prosthodont 2009;22(3):251–9.

46. Meyer RA. The temporomandibular joint examination. In: Walker HK, Hall WD, Hurst JW, editors. Clinical methods: the history, physical, and laboratory examinations. 3rd edition. Boston: Butterworths; 1990. p. 763–4. Available at: http://www.ncbi.nlm.nih.gov/books/NBK271/.

47. Ramar K, Dort LC, Katz SG, et al. Clinical practice guideline for the treatment of obstructive sleep apnea and snoring with oral appliance therapy: an update for 2015. J Clin Sleep Med 2015;11(7):773–827.

48. Maimon N, Hanly PJ. Does snoring intensity correlate with the severity of obstructive sleep apnea? J Clin Sleep Med 2010;6(5):475–8.

49. American Academy of Sleep Medicine/American Academy of Dental Sleep Medicine. Policy statement on the diagnosis and treatment of obstructive sleep apnea. 2012. Available at: http://www.aasmnet.org/resources/pdf/AADSM JointOSApolicy.pdf. Accessed March 13, 2016.

50. Hoffstein V. Review of oral appliances for treatment of sleep-disordered breathing. Sleep Breath 2007;11(1):1–22.

51. American Academy of Dental Sleep Medicine. AADSM treatment protocol: oral appliance therapy for sleep disordered breathing: an update for 2013. 2013. Available at: http://www.aadsm.org/treatmentprotocol.aspx. Accessed March 14, 2016.

52. American Academy of Dental Sleep Medicine. AADSM protocol for oral appliance therapy for sleep disordered breathing in adults: an update for 2012. 2012. Available at: http://www.aadsm.org/PDFs/TreatmentProtocolOAT.pdf. Accessed March 14, 2016.

# Drug-Induced Sleep Endoscopy

Natamon Charakorn, MD[a],*, Eric J. Kezirian, MD, MPH[b]

## KEYWORDS

- Obstructive sleep apnea • Drug-induced sleep endoscopy • Snoring • Surgery

## KEY POINTS

- Drug-induced sleep endoscopy (DISE) is an upper airway evaluation technique with 3 key features: the use of pharmacologic agents to achieve sedation, the target depth of sedation as approximating natural sleep as much as possible, and the endoscopic evaluation of the upper airway.
- The VOTE Classification incorporates the 4 major structures that contribute to airway obstruction in most patients: Velum (palate), Oropharyngeal lateral walls, Tongue, and Epiglottis.
- DISE may improve treatment selection in sleep-disordered breathing, especially in patients with obstructive sleep apnea unable to tolerate positive airway pressure therapy.

## INTRODUCTION

Because up to 50% of patients with obstructive sleep apnea (OSA) are unable to tolerate positive airway pressure therapy,[1] alternative treatments, such as surgery, upper airway stimulation, or oral appliances, may be required. Comprehensive patient evaluation is a key to success for the latter group of treatments. The goal of evaluation is to determine the pattern of airway obstruction, with the ultimate aim of designing targeted, effective treatment.

The ideal evaluation technique would be an assessment of breathing, sleeping patients, as this would provide a real-time, dynamic assessment. It would also be safe, noninvasive, and low cost. The desire to directly visualize airway obstruction led some investigators to perform fiberoptic examination during natural sleep in the late 1970s and early 1980s.[2,3] However, these efforts were generally abandoned due to the

Disclosures: None.
a Department of Otolaryngology - Head and Neck Surgery, Faculty of Medicine, Chulalongkorn University and King Chulalonkorn Memorial Hospital, Thai Red Cross Society, 1873 Rama 4 Road, Patumwan, Bangkok 10330, Thailand; b USC Caruso Department of Otolaryngology - Head and Neck Surgery, Keck School of Medicine of USC, 1450 San Pablo Street, Suite 5100, Los Angeles, CA 90033, USA
* Corresponding author.
E-mail address: natamonc@gmail.com

discomfort experience by patients, particularly with movement of the endoscope to view multiple areas of the pharyngeal airway.

Fiberoptic evaluation of the upper airway under conditions of sedation was developed in a number of centers in Europe in the late 1980s, and Croft and Pringle[4] first described their technique of "sleep nasendoscopy" in 1991. The nomenclature was changed to "drug-induced sleep endoscopy" (DISE) by Kezirian and Hohenhorst (W. Hohenhorst, personal communication, 2005) to reflect the 3 key features of this method: the potential use of various pharmacologic agents to achieve sedation, the target depth of sedation as approximating natural sleep as much as possible, and the endoscopic evaluation of the upper airway. In contrast to other procedures that usually provide 2-dimensional assessments during wakefulness in the upright sitting position, DISE provides a 3-dimensional evaluation of the airway during unconscious sedation.

This article presents recommendations regarding DISE technique and reviews the evidence concerning the role of DISE in the evaluation of OSA.

## TECHNIQUE
### Indications/Contraindications

Any diagnostic evaluation will be useful if the benefits outweigh the risks. For DISE, the benefits include potential value in treatment selection, and the risks are related to the sedative agent used and the potential for significant airway compromise. Indications and contraindications are listed in **Box 1**.

### Sedative Agent

Control of the depth of sedation is essential. The sedative agent will generally be administered intravenously at the minimum dose to achieve the target depth of sedation: the loss of consciousness, defined as loss of response to verbal stimulation at a

---

**Box 1**
**Indication and contraindication for drug-induced sleep endoscopy**

*Indications*

Patients with obstructive sleep apnea (OSA) (or snoring, in some countries)

Unable to tolerate positive airway pressure (in countries in which positive airway pressure is the first-line treatment modality for OSA)

Consideration of surgery, oral appliances, positional therapy, or combination approaches

*Contraindications (relative)*

Allergy to sedative agents

Pregnancy

Significant medical comorbidities

Optional contraindications used by some surgeons:
  Markedly severe OSA (AHI >70 events per hour)
  Obesity (body mass index >35 kg/m$^2$)

normal conversational volume, similar to a modified Ramsay score of 5.[5] Multiple sedative agents have been used as effective agents in the performance of DISE. The commonly used sedative agents included propofol, midazolam, propofol with midazolam, and dexmedetomidine. Pharmacologic properties of these sedative agents is shown in **Table 1**.

The choice of sedative agent, to some extent, depends on its ability to reproduce some of the changes that occur in natural sleep. During sleep, upper airway patency relies on pharyngeal dilator muscle tone and changes in lung volume that counteract collapsing forces, principally intraluminal negative pressure generated during inspiration and anatomic narrowing of the airway.[6] Patients with OSA maintain pharyngeal patency with greater dilator (genioglossus) muscle tone during wakefulness, but sleep onset results in marked decreases in muscle tone due to the loss of the wakefulness stimulus and decreases in negative pressure reflex activity and lung volume.[7-13] Rapid eye movement (REM) sleep has greater reductions in muscle tone and lung volumes than non-REM (NREM) sleep.[9-13] The continuum of sedation ranges from wakefulness to conscious sedation to unconscious sedation to general anesthesia, in which arousability to all stimulation is lost. Deeper levels of sedation are associated with progressive decreases in upper airway dilator muscle tone and neuromuscular reflex activation, both of which increase airway collapsibility.[9,11-15]

Unconscious sedation represents a lesser degree of neural depression than anesthesia and may be a closer approximation to natural sleep. The interest in the transition from wakefulness to unconscious sedation is based on the concept of a thalamocortical switch determining consciousness or unconsciousness (no response to verbal stimulation) that may be common to natural sleep and sedation.[16,17]

Propofol can be administered with target-controlled infusion, continuous infusion, or using small boluses. The most-detailed study of changes in upper airway physiology associated with propofol sedation had results consistent with the thalamocortical switch described previously, as changes in upper airway collapsibility (passive Pcrit), Bispectral Index Score (based on frontal electroencephalogram activity), and muscle tone occurred at this transition from consciousness to unconsciousness disproportionate to changes in propofol concentration.[14] During propofol unconscious sedation, healthy individuals have decreases in genioglossus tone to 10% of

**Table 1**
**Pharmacologic properties of propofol, midazolam, and dexmedetomidine**

|  | Propofol | Midazolam | Dexmedetomidine |
|---|---|---|---|
| Sedative agents | 2-6-diisopropylphenol | Benzodiazepine | Alpha-2 adrenergic receptor agonist |
| Functional half-life | 4–6 min | 45 min | 6 min |
| Elimination half-life | 3 h | 150 min | 2 h |
| Accumulation | Inactive metabolite (no accumulation) | Active metabolite (alpha-hydroxymidazolam) | Inactive metabolite (no accumulation) |
| Therapeutic range | Small | Large | Small |
| Respiratory side effects (potential) | Respiratory depression and hypopharyngeal reflex depression | Respiratory depression | None |
| Cardiovascular side effects (potential) | Hypotension | Hypotension | Fluctuation of blood pressure and heart rate |

maximum awake activity,[14,18] which is one-half to one-third of the level in NREM sleep in healthy individuals,[8] but greater than during REM sleep in healthy individuals and patients with OSA.[19]

To achieve this depth of sedation, target-controlled infusion with the Diprifusor (Astra-Zeneca, Inc, London, United Kingdom) technology is available in many countries, using a proprietary algorithm to achieve effect site (brain) concentration using a 3-compartment pharmacokinetic model.[18,20] This technology is not available in the United States and many other countries, so some surgeons use a protocol involving continuous infusion (usually unconscious sedation requires 100–150 μg/kg per minute), with possible additional boluses (eg, 20–50 mg). Other surgeons prefer using a continuous infusion without administration of boluses. It is important that different individuals can require markedly different dosages of propofol to reach the target depth of sedation.[14,21]

Dexmedetomidine has been used extensively in anesthesia for a wide range of procedures and for prolonged periods of sedation, with comparable performance during general anesthesia.[22] As is true for midazolam, there has been no study evaluating the impact of dexmedetomidine on upper airway muscle tone and airway collapsibility.

Dexmedetomidine may achieve a depth of anesthesia comparable to propofol for general surgical procedures,[22] but in one study, half of the patients required supplemental propofol during drug-induced sleep endoscopy because they did not achieve adequate sedation despite a maximum dose of dexmedetomidine (1.4 μg/kg/h).[23] The senior author (Dr Kezirian) has seen a number of patients who underwent DISE using dexmedetomidine at other institutions in which there was no airway obstruction visualized despite apparent loss of consciousness; this may reflect a lesser decrease in upper airway muscle tone with dexmedetomidine compared with propofol and midazolam, but there are no data evaluating this to date.

### Preoperative Preparation

Preoperative anesthetics other than the sedative agent of choice should be avoided. To prevent regurgitation and aspiration, patients should remain nil per os (NPO) before the procedure. Anticholinergic agents, such as atropine or glycopyrrolate, can be administered intravenously 30 minutes before the procedure to reduce secretions, leading to better visualization and avoidance of coughing due to aspiration during the procedure; mild tachycardia is commonly observed with these anticholinergic agents.

A topical vasoconstrictor is generally applied to 1 or both nostrils, and topical anesthetic is applied to 1 nostril. The dose of topical anesthetic is minimized to avoid excessive pharyngeal anesthesia that can lead to coughing during the procedure (again, due to aspiration of secretions) or blunting of muscular reflexes that promote upper airway patency.[24] Awake fiberoptic examination performed before initiating sedation can confirm adequate topical anesthesia. This awake examination also allows the anesthesia team the opportunity to visualize the airway before administration of sedation to a patient with sleep-disordered breathing, often providing some additional level of comfort.

Surgeon preferences regarding patient positioning vary widely. Some prefer to use the supine position in all patients, as this body position is used by many patients for at least a portion of the night and may reflect the body position that is most problematic for OSA. Other surgeons prefer to use the patient's natural body position during sleep. Still others evaluate the patient in both the lateral and supine positions or turn the head to the side while the trunk is in the supine position.[25] There is no single best approach, but if possible the surgeon should examine the body (or head) position that will provide the greatest amount of information to use in treatment selection.

### Setting and Monitoring

DISE is usually performed in the operating room or procedure suite, but it is also possible to perform DISE in various outpatient settings, depending on the availability of personnel and appropriate equipment for administering sedation safely. The temperature of the room should be set as comfortable as possible. Lights should be dimmed, and the room noise should be minimized.

Oxygen saturation, cardiac rhythm, and blood pressure monitoring are required during the procedure. Supplemental oxygen may not be necessary, but it should be available for potential use. Some surgeons prefer routine administration of oxygen via nasal cannula or face mask placed on the upper chest in a "blow-by" fashion.

The most important evaluation of the depth of sedation is clinical, through the onset of snoring, disordered breathing events, and the loss of consciousness. Bispectral index (BIS) score may provide additional monitoring of sedation.[14] BIS score is associated with the depth of sedation, with a potential target BIS score of 55 to 70, based on changes in muscle tone and upper airway collapsibility.[14] Greater depth of sedation may produce greater loss of muscle tone and increased airway collapsibility. One study of DISE using propofol showed an increase in airway obstruction (both severity and contribution of the palate and tongue) at BIS scores of 50 to 60 versus 65 to 75.[26]

### Risks and Disadvantages

No catastrophic events have been reported with DISE. Endotracheal intubation is extremely rare, and cricothyrotomy and tracheostomy also have not been reported. Oversedation that may lead to airway compromise or central apnea can be prevented by titrating the sedative agent to the lowest level that maintains the target of sedation. Supplemental oxygen or concurrent positive airway pressure administration may be an option to prevent complications in high-risk patients, such as those with morbid obesity or greater medical comorbidity. Other DISE risks include local pain on intravenous infusion of propofol and allergic reaction to medications.

## DIAGNOSIS
### Airway Evaluation: The VOTE Classification

DISE is principally an examination of the pharynx, and during the examination, the flexible fiberoptic laryngoscope is moved a number of times to evaluate the entire length of the pharynx across a number of cycles of airway obstruction and normal breathing.[27] A surgeon must recognize that they are often visualizing only a portion of the pharynx at a single point in time, necessitating evaluation and reevaluation of different regions to understand, to the extent possible, the source(s) of airway obstruction over a period of time in different body positions, during various maneuvers, and so forth.

A variety of classification schemes have been described to characterize DISE findings. There are at least 7 schemes reported in the literature, with a wide range of complexity.[4,27–32] The VOTE Classification was proposed as a standard for DISE scoring because it incorporates the 4 major structures that contribute to airway obstruction in most patients: Velum (palate), Oropharyngeal lateral walls, Tongue, and Epiglottis. The hope is that widespread adoption of the VOTE Classification would lead to the sharing of findings and results across centers, enhancing clinical and research communication and collaboration.

### The Structures of the VOTE Acronym

The VOTE Classification allows a surgeon to characterize the structures that contribute to pharyngeal obstruction in a patient, incorporating the degree and configuration of airway narrowing related to these structures that are each composed of multiple components.

### Velum

Velum-related obstruction is that related to the palate and occurs due to the soft palate, uvula, or lateral pharyngeal wall tissue at the level of the velopharynx. Airway closure related to the velum can occur with collapse in an anteroposterior (**Fig. 1**), concentric, or, less commonly, lateral configuration. Because it is not always possible to distinguish between the soft palate, uvula, and lateral pharyngeal walls at the level of the velopharynx on DISE, the VOTE Classification groups them under the umbrella of the Velum. The lateral pharyngeal walls at the level of the velopharynx have some interaction with the remainder of the lateral wall tissues, but in the VOTE Classification, there is an attempt to describe these separately.

### Oropharyngeal lateral walls, including tonsils

The oropharyngeal lateral walls include the palatine tonsils and the lateral pharyngeal wall tissues that include muscles and the adjacent parapharyngeal fat pads, among other elements. In the VOTE Classification, the oropharyngeal lateral walls collapse only in a lateral configuration (**Fig. 2**), although there can be some collapse of tissues originating on the posterior pharyngeal walls that create the impression of a concentric pattern. In the presence of lateral wall collapse, it can be difficult (but certainly not impossible) to determine whether the tonsils alone are the source of airway obstruction or whether the other lateral pharyngeal tissues also contribute. The distinction can have important implications for treatment selection and outcomes. Although the VOTE Classification is largely based on DISE findings alone, the examination of tonsil size and lateral pharyngeal wall tissues during routine oral cavity examination can be invaluable in making a determination of potential contributions of each of these structural elements.

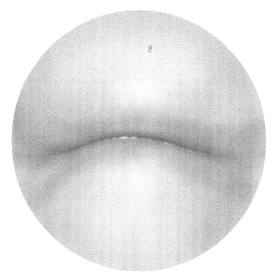

**Fig. 1.** Velum obstruction in an anteroposterior configuration.

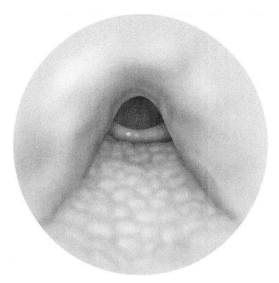

**Fig. 2.** Oropharyngeal lateral walls collapse in a lateral configuration.

### Tongue

Tongue-related obstruction is a common DISE finding, and it results in anteroposterior narrowing of the upper airway (**Fig. 3**). In natural sleep, there is a reduction in upper airway muscle tone. Because the tongue is largely composed of muscle and fat, this muscle relaxation leads to tongue-related airway obstruction in many patients. Tongue-related obstruction occurs in an anteroposterior configuration only.

### Epiglottis

Epiglottic collapse may occur in an anteroposterior (**Fig. 4**) or lateral configuration. Anteroposterior collapse can result with folding of the epiglottis based on what

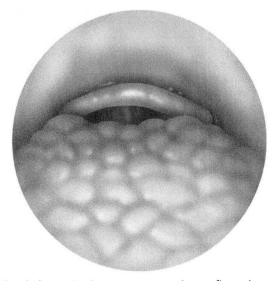

**Fig. 3.** Tongue-related obstruction in an anteroposterior configuration.

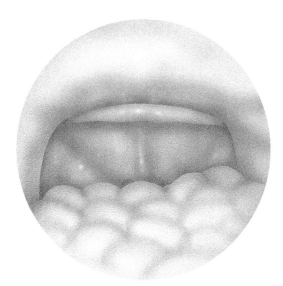

**Fig. 4.** Epiglottic collapse in an anteroposterior configuration.

appears to be decreased structural rigidity of the epiglottis or with a posterior displacement of the entire epiglottis against the posterior pharyngeal wall, with apparently normal epiglottic structural integrity. In the rarer lateral collapse, a lateral folding or involution is consistent with a central vertically oriented crease of decreased rigidity of the epiglottis. The epiglottis may be underrecognized as a factor in patients with sleep-disordered breathing, and a substantial proportion of patients with OSA demonstrate a significant epiglottic contribution to airway obstruction during DISE.[21,33] Identifying epiglottic contribution is unique to DISE, as its apparent role has not been demonstrated clearly with other evaluation techniques.[34,35]

### Other Structures

Airway obstruction in sleep-disordered breathing can be related to other structures. In rare cases, collapse superior to the VOTE structures (eg, massive nasal polyps or nasopharynx) or inferior to the VOTE structures (eg, larynx) can be visualized. These are usually detected by awake examination before DISE and are noted separately. Although these are important, the VOTE Classification was developed to reflect the patterns of pharyngeal obstruction seen in the large majority of patients.

### Degree of Airway Narrowing

The VOTE Classification involves a qualitative assessment of the degree of airway narrowing for each structure, divided into the following:

  *None* (typically with no vibration of the involved structure and <50% airway narrowing compared with dimensions during spontaneous breathing);

  *Partial* (vibration, 50%–75% narrowing, possible reduced airflow); or

  *Complete* (obstruction, >75% narrowing, markedly reduced or absent airflow).

Differentiating among the 3 categories is not always clear, although as outlined in this article, the evaluation of degree of obstruction has demonstrated moderate to substantial reliability.[21,36] Importantly, different structures can have different degrees (and configuration) of obstruction in the same patient.

The VOTE Classification does not exclude additional assessments. DISE can be performed in various body positions, as described previously. If there are differential patterns of obstruction according to body position, this may require separate VOTE scoring for each body position.

DISE permits certain maneuvers, ranging from manual closure of the mouth only to the Esmarch maneuver (mandibular advancement). Open-mouth breathing is associated with reduction of the retropalatal and retroglossal areas, thus can worsen OSA.[37] One-third of patients with persistent OSA after previous palate surgery have moderate to severe mouth opening, with half demonstrating marked improvement in airway obstruction with manual mouth closure during DISE.[38] The Esmarch maneuver is performed by gently advancing the mandible by up to approximately 5 mm, in an attempt to reproduce the effect of a mandibular repositioning appliance. Other techniques are available for this purpose.[39] As for differences according to body position, multiple separate VOTE assessments can be used during a single DISE to record changes in the pattern of collapse that occur after an assessment with these maneuvers.

## CLINICAL OUTCOMES
### Test Properties of Drug-Induced Sleep Endoscopy: Validity, Reliability, and Uniqueness of Information

Any useful diagnostic test must demonstrate key characteristics, such as validity and reliability, and these have been examined for DISE.

DISE is not a perfect representation of natural sleep. Nevertheless, light sedation with relatively low doses of propofol using target-controlled infusion did not produce marked changes in the apnea-hypopnea index or oxygen saturations, compared with natural sleep.[40]

Administration of propofol at a wide range of doses that were relatively high at the maximum levels did not cause any snoring or airway obstruction in 54 subjects without a history of snoring or witnessed apneas, whereas all 53 subjects with such a history demonstrated snoring and/or airway obstruction.[41] Another study showed greater airway collapsibility in those with OSA compared with those with primary snoring during sedation with propofol.[42]

Interrater reliability reflects the degree to which ratings from different reviewers are similar. Interrater reliability was moderate to substantial in one study of 2 experienced reviewers,[21] and another study showed greater interrater reliability for experienced versus nonexperienced reviewers.[43] Test-retest reliability evaluates the ratings on distinct DISE examinations performed on the same patient. Test-retest reliability also has been shown to be moderate to substantial.[36] This is in sharp contrast to the marked variation seen among different patients undergoing DISE,[33] a reassuring finding that likely relates to the heterogeneity of anatomic factors contributing to OSA.

Information taken from DISE is different from other upper airway evaluation techniques. No association was seen between elevated modified Mallampati score (reflecting a tongue size that is large relative to space posterior to the mandible) and tongue-related obstruction during DISE performed with propofol.[34] Another study compared findings of DISE performed with propofol and the lateral cephalogram radiograph. Amid an extensive series of measurements, only the posterior airway space (anteroposterior dimension of the airway posterior to the tongue base) was associated with tongue-related obstruction.[35]

## Drug-Induced Sleep Endoscopy and Airway Surgery

Because the purpose of DISE is guiding treatment selection, the most important clinical questions may relate to the association between DISE findings and outcomes of various interventions. Multiple studies have examined such questions, in addition to one study suggesting that DISE may alter treatment recommendations in 78% of cases.[44]

Subjects with anteroposterior palate-related obstruction or obstruction related to the palatine tonsils on DISE performed with diazepam achieved better outcome after uvulopalatopharyngoplasty (with tonsillectomy in those without previous tonsillectomy) than those with concentric palate-related obstruction or obstruction related to structures other than the palate or tonsils (with or without palate-related or tonsil-related obstruction).[31] Similarly, patients with nasal and palatal obstruction during DISE performed with propofol had better outcomes after uvulopalatopharyngoplasty than those with hypopharyngeal region obtsruction.[45]

Preoperative findings of DISE performed with propofol also have been associated with surgical outcomes in cohort studies involving single-level and multilevel surgery. Among a group of patients undergoing a range of procedures (including nasal surgery, uvulopalatopharyngoplasty, the Pillar Procedure, genioglossus advancement, tongue base resection, tongue stabilization, and hyoid suspension) that resulted in a 56% response rate ($\geq$50% reduction in apnea-hypopnea index to <20 events per hour), preoperative DISE findings of complete oropharyngeal lateral wall–related obstruction and complete epiglottis-related obstruction were associated with nonresponse to surgery.[46] Another study involving DISE performed with propofol included those undergoing 1 or more procedures from among uvulopalatopharyngoplasty, Z-palatoplasty, tongue base radiofrequency, and hyoid suspension; individuals with complete concentric collapse of the velum or complete tongue-related obstruction had poorer outcomes, after adjusting for age, gender, apnea-hypopnea index, and body mass index.[47]

DISE also has been used to examine nonresponders to single-level or multilevel pharyngeal OSA surgery. DISE performed with propofol revealed a wide range of potential sources of residual airway obstruction, including that related to the velum or other VOTE structures and moderate to severe mouth opening that was associated with narrowing of upper airway dimensions.[38]

## Drug-Induced Sleep Endoscopy and Hypoglossal Nerve Stimulation

Hypoglossal nerve stimulation has been introduced recently as a treatment modality. In an early study of one technology, complete concentric collapse of the velum during DISE performed with propofol was associated with poorer outcomes: 0% (0/5) versus 81% (13/16) response rate, based on a definition of response of 50% or more decrease in apnea-hypopnea index to less than 20 events per hour.[48] This study led to the use of DISE in patient selection for the major trial of this technology[49] and the requirement of DISE in patient selection for clinical use in the United States. A study performed at the completion of this trial revealed that, during DISE performed with an individual in the supine body position, this technology produced an overall 180% enlargement of the cross-sectional area of the retropalatal airway and 130% increase in the cross-sectional area of the hypopharyngeal region airway.[50] Interestingly, the increase in retropalatal airway cross-sectional area was limited to the anteroposterior dimension, whereas there was enlargement of the transverse and anteroposterior dimensions in the hypopharyngeal region airway.

## Nonsurgical Approaches

Because positional OSA is so common, it is interesting to note the changes that have been demonstrated with changes in body position during DISE. Sleep position has been shown to alter the pattern of obstruction during DISE in individuals with positional (but not nonpositional) OSA.[51] The supine body position was associated with a greater presence and severity of obstruction related to the tongue and epiglottis in positional OSA. In another study, head turning to the side (with body in the supine position) produced findings similar to those with the head and body both in the lateral position, with the exception of greater anteroposterior velum-related obstruction with the head and body both in the lateral position.[25] This suggests that head rotation may be a reasonable substitute, facilitating the assessment of positional therapy.

The Esmarch maneuver during DISE may indicate benefit of treatment with a mandibular repositioning appliance. Among patients with OSA who showed a substantial improvement in airway dimensions with mandibular advancement during DISE performed with propofol, 97% achieved an improvement in subjective or objective measures (not defined clearly) with mandibular repositioning appliance treatment.[52] Another study from the same group showed that DISE performed with propofol with the patient wearing the mandibular repositioning device achieves changes in the airway similar to manual mandibular advancement.[53] Manual mandibular advancement may produce arousals and may not capture the degree of mouth opening that occurs with a mandibular repositioning appliance, it is possible to use a custom-fabricated mouthpiece to simulate the effect of mandibular advancement.[39]

## SUMMARY

Identifying the pattern of airway obstruction in OSA is critical. No single ideal method exists, although DISE is an attractive option. DISE is a structure-based surgical evaluation technique that may enable targeted, more effective, and less-invasive treatment of snoring and OSA.

## REFERENCES

1. Weaver TE, Grunstein RR. Adherence to continuous positive airway pressure therapy: the challenge to effective treatment. Proc Am Thorac Soc 2008;5:173–8.
2. Borowiecki B, Pollak CP, Weitzman ED, et al. Fibro-optic study of pharyngeal airway during sleep in patients with hypersomnia obstructive sleep-apnea syndrome. Laryngoscope 1978;88:1310–3.
3. Rojewski TE, Schuller DE, Clark RW, et al. Synchronous video recording of the pharyngeal airway and polysomnograph in patients with obstructive sleep apnea. Laryngoscope 1982;92:246–50.
4. Croft CB, Pringle M. Sleep nasendoscopy: a technique of assessment in snoring and obstructive sleep apnoea. Clin Otolaryngol Allied Sci 1991;16:504–9.
5. Ramsay MA, Savege TM, Simpson BR, et al. Controlled sedation with alphaxalone-alphadolone. Br Med J 1974;2:656–9.
6. White DP. Pathogenesis of obstructive and central sleep apnea. Am J Respir Crit Care Med 2005;172:1363–70.
7. Fogel RB, Trinder J, Malhotra A, et al. Within-breath control of genioglossal muscle activation in humans: effect of sleep-wake state. J Physiol 2003;550:899–910.
8. Fogel RB, Trinder J, White DP, et al. The effect of sleep onset on upper airway muscle activity in patients with sleep apnoea versus controls. J Physiol 2005; 564:549–62.

9. Horner RL, Innes JA, Morrell MJ, et al. The effect of sleep on reflex genioglossus muscle activation by stimuli of negative airway pressure in humans. J Physiol 1994;476:141–51.

10. Malhotra A, Pillar G, Fogel RB, et al. Genioglossal but not palatal muscle activity relates closely to pharyngeal pressure. Am J Respir Crit Care Med 2000;162: 1058–62.

11. Shea SA, Edwards JK, White DP. Effects of sleep-wake transitions and REM sleep on genioglossal response to upper airway negative pressure. Am J Respir Crit Care Med 1998;157:A653.

12. Wheatley JR, Tangel DJ, Mezzanotte WS, et al. Influence of sleep on response to negative airway pressure of tensor palatini muscle and retropalatal airway. J Appl Physiol (1985) 1993;75:2117–24.

13. Wheatley JR, White DP. The influence of sleep on pharyngeal reflexes. Sleep 1993;16:S87–9.

14. Hillman DR, Walsh JH, Maddison KJ, et al. Evolution of changes in upper airway collapsibility during slow induction of anesthesia with propofol. Anesthesiology 2009;111:63–71.

15. Tangel DJ, Mezzanotte WS, White DP. Influence of sleep on tensor palatini EMG and upper airway resistance in normal men. J Appl Physiol (1985) 1991;70: 2574–81.

16. Alkire MT, Haier RJ, Fallon JH. Toward a unified theory of narcosis: brain imaging evidence for a thalamocortical switch as the neurophysiologic basis of anesthetic-induced unconsciousness. Conscious Cogn 2000;9:370–86.

17. Saper CB, Chou TC, Scammell TE. The sleep switch: hypothalamic control of sleep and wakefulness. Trends Neurosci 2001;24:726–31.

18. Eastwood PR, Platt PR, Shepherd K, et al. Collapsibility of the upper airway at different concentrations of propofol anesthesia. Anesthesiology 2005;103:470–7.

19. Eckert DJ, Malhotra A, Lo YL, et al. The influence of obstructive sleep apnea and gender on genioglossus activity during rapid eye movement sleep. Chest 2009; 135:957–64.

20. Roblin G, Williams AR, Whittet H. Target-controlled infusion in sleep endoscopy. Laryngoscope 2001;111:175–6.

21. Kezirian EJ, White DP, Malhotra A, et al. Interrater reliability of drug-induced sleep endoscopy. Arch Otolaryngol Head Neck Surg 2010;136:393–7.

22. Chattopadhyay U, Mallik S, Ghosh S, et al. Comparison between propofol and dexmedetomidine on depth of anesthesia: a prospective randomized trial. J Anaesthesiol Clin Pharmacol 2014;30:550–4.

23. Cho JS, Soh S, Kim EJ, et al. Comparison of three sedation regimens for drug-induced sleep endoscopy. Sleep Breath 2015;19:711–7.

24. Fogel RB, Malhotra A, Shea SA, et al. Reduced genioglossal activity with upper airway anesthesia in awake patients with OSA. J Appl Physiol (1985) 2000;88: 1346–54.

25. Safiruddin F, Koutsourelakis I, de Vries N. Upper airway collapse during drug induced sleep endoscopy: head rotation in supine position compared with lateral head and trunk position. Eur Arch Otorhinolaryngol 2015;272:485–8.

26. Lo YL, Ni YL, Wang TY, et al. Bispectral index in evaluating effects of sedation depth on drug-induced sleep endoscopy. J Clin Sleep Med 2015;11(9):1011–20.

27. Kezirian EJ, Hohenhorst W, de Vries N. Drug-induced sleep endoscopy: the VOTE classification. Eur Arch Otorhinolaryngol 2011;268:1233–6.

28. Abdullah VJ, Wing YK, van Hasselt CA. Video sleep nasendoscopy: the Hong Kong experience. Otolaryngol Clin North Am 2003;36:461–71, vi.

29. Friedman M, Ibrahim H, Bass L. Clinical staging for sleep-disordered breathing. Otolaryngol Head Neck Surg 2002;127:13–21.
30. Fujita S, Conway W, Zorick F, et al. Surgical correction of anatomic abnormalities in obstructive sleep apnea syndrome: uvulopalatopharyngoplasty. Otolaryngol Head Neck Surg 1981;89:923–34.
31. Iwanaga K, Hasegawa K, Shibata N, et al. Endoscopic examination of obstructive sleep apnea syndrome patients during drug-induced sleep. Acta Otolaryngol Suppl 2003;550:36–40.
32. Vicini C, De Vito A, Benazzo M, et al. The nose oropharynx hypopharynx and larynx (NOHL) classification: a new system of diagnostic standardized examination for OSAHS patients. Eur Arch Otorhinolaryngol 2012;269:1297–300.
33. Vroegop AV, Vanderveken OM, Boudewyns AN, et al. Drug-induced sleep endoscopy in sleep-disordered breathing: report on 1,249 cases. Laryngoscope 2014; 124:797–802.
34. den Herder C, van Tinteren H, de Vries N. Sleep endoscopy versus modified Mallampati score in sleep apnea and snoring. Laryngoscope 2005;115:735–9.
35. George JR, Chung S, Nielsen I, et al. Comparison of drug-induced sleep endoscopy and lateral cephalometry in obstructive sleep apnea. Laryngoscope 2012; 122:2600–5.
36. Rodriguez-Bruno K, Goldberg AN, McCulloch CE, et al. Test-retest reliability of drug-induced sleep endoscopy. Otolaryngol Head Neck Surg 2009;140:646–51.
37. Lee CH, Hong SL, Rhee CS, et al. Analysis of upper airway obstruction by sleep videofluoroscopy in obstructive sleep apnea: a large population-based study. Laryngoscope 2012;122:237–41.
38. Kezirian EJ. Nonresponders to pharyngeal surgery for obstructive sleep apnea: insights from drug-induced sleep endoscopy. Laryngoscope 2011;121:1320–6.
39. Vroegop AV, Vanderveken OM, Dieltjens M, et al. Sleep endoscopy with simulation bite for prediction of oral appliance treatment outcome. J Sleep Res 2013; 22:348–55.
40. Rabelo FA, Braga A, Kupper DS, et al. Propofol-induced sleep: polysomnographic evaluation of patients with obstructive sleep apnea and controls. Otolaryngol Head Neck Surg 2010;142:218–24.
41. Berry S, Roblin G, Williams A, et al. Validity of sleep nasendoscopy in the investigation of sleep related breathing disorders. Laryngoscope 2005;115:538–40.
42. Steinhart H, Kuhn-Lohmann J, Gewalt K, et al. Upper airway collapsibility in habitual snorers and sleep apneics: evaluation with drug-induced sleep endoscopy. Acta Otolaryngol 2000;120:990–4.
43. Vroegop AV, Vanderveken OM, Wouters K, et al. Observer variation in drug-induced sleep endoscopy: experienced versus nonexperienced ear, nose, and throat surgeons. Sleep 2013;36:947–53.
44. Eichler C, Sommer JU, Stuck BA, et al. Does drug-induced sleep endoscopy change the treatment concept of patients with snoring and obstructive sleep apnea? Sleep Breath 2013;17:63–8.
45. Hessel NS, Vries N. Increase of the apnoea-hypopnoea index after uvulopalatopharyngoplasty: analysis of failure. Clin Otolaryngol Allied Sci 2004;29:682–5.
46. Soares D, Sinawe H, Folbe AJ, et al. Lateral oropharyngeal wall and supraglottic airway collapse associated with failure in sleep apnea surgery. Laryngoscope 2012;122:473–9.
47. Koutsourelakis I, Safiruddin F, Ravesloot M, et al. Surgery for obstructive sleep apnea: sleep endoscopy determinants of outcome. Laryngoscope 2012;122: 2587–91.

48. Vanderveken OM, Maurer JT, Hohenhorst W, et al. Evaluation of drug-induced sleep endoscopy as a patient selection tool for implanted upper airway stimulation for obstructive sleep apnea. J Clin Sleep Med 2013;9:433–8.
49. Strollo PJ Jr, Soose RJ, Maurer JT, et al. Upper-airway stimulation for obstructive sleep apnea. N Engl J Med 2014;370:139–49.
50. Safiruddin F, Vanderveken OM, de Vries N, et al. Effect of upper-airway stimulation for obstructive sleep apnoea on airway dimensions. Eur Respir J 2015;45:129–38.
51. Victores AJ, Hamblin J, Gilbert J, et al. Usefulness of sleep endoscopy in predicting positional obstructive sleep apnea. Otolaryngol Head Neck Surg 2014;150:487–93.
52. Johal A, Battagel JM, Kotecha BT. Sleep nasendoscopy: a diagnostic tool for predicting treatment success with mandibular advancement splints in obstructive sleep apnoea. Eur J Orthod 2005;27:607–14.
53. Johal A, Hector MP, Battagel JM, et al. Impact of sleep nasendoscopy on the outcome of mandibular advancement splint therapy in subjects with sleep-related breathing disorders. J Laryngol Otol 2007;121:668–75.

# Nasal Surgery for Obstructive Sleep Apnea Syndrome

 CrossMark

Samuel A. Mickelson, MD, FACS, FABSM

## KEYWORDS

- Nasal obstruction • Nasal surgery • Septoplasty • Turbinate reduction
- Obstructive sleep apnea syndrome • Sleep disordered breathing
- CPAP compliance

## KEY POINTS

- Mechanical and inflammatory factors leading to nasal obstruction contribute to sleep disordered breathing by increasing nasal airway resistance, causing sleep fragmentation, and causing mouth breathing.
- Treatment of obstructive sleep apnea with continuous positive airway pressure (CPAP) is considered the first line of therapy, but long-term compliance is only about 40%, often because of nasal obstruction.
- Medical treatment with topical nasal steroid sprays and nasal dilators have been shown to improve sleep disordered breathing.
- Surgical treatment of nasal obstruction, including septoplasty, turbinate reduction, and nasal valve reconstruction, has been shown to improve sleep disordered breathing.
- Surgical treatment of nasal obstruction has been shown to reduce CPAP requirement and improve compliance with CPAP.

## OVERVIEW OF OBSTRUCTIVE SLEEP APNEA

Obstructive sleep apnea (OSA) is a major health problem in the United States. With a prevalence in middle-aged adults of 2% to 4%[1] of the population, untreated OSA has been implicated in increased risk for cardiovascular disease, including hypertension and heart failure.[2–7]

The standard test for diagnosis of OSA is polysomnography, which produces outputs on several physiologic variables. The apnea-hypopnea index (AHI), expressed as the number of apneas and hypopneas per hour of sleep, and respiratory

Disclosures: Research funding from Inspire Medical Inc, Imthera Medical Inc. Consultant for Zelegent Inc, Siesta Medical Inc.
Advanced Ear Nose & Throat Associates, The Atlanta Snoring & Sleep Disorders Institute, 960 Johnson Ferry Road Northeast, Suite 200, Atlanta, GA 30342, USA
E-mail address: sam@advancedENTpc.com

Otolaryngol Clin N Am 49 (2016) 1373–1381
http://dx.doi.org/10.1016/j.otc.2016.07.002
0030-6665/16/© 2016 Elsevier Inc. All rights reserved.

disturbance index (RDI), expressed as the number of apneas, hypopneas, and respiratory effort–related arousals per hour of sleep are the most important reported measures of disease severity. In general, an AHI or RDI of 5 or greater connotes a diagnosis of sleep apnea, 5 to 14 is defined as mild disease, 15 to 29 as moderate disease, and 30 or greater as severe disease. The goal of treatment of OSA is improvement in quality of life and longevity. Secondary outcome measures include a reduction of AHI and RDI and other key variables, such as lowest oxygen saturation, (LSAT) or oxygen desaturation index (ODI) as measured on polysomnography.

The first-line and most common treatment of OSA is positive airway pressure (PAP) treatment. PAP is effective in reducing the AHI and RDI if used properly. However, the mask interface, air pressure required, and need to use a machine at the bedside all night lead to poor acceptance and compliance rates. Compliance with PAP was defined by Kribbs and colleagues[8] as using PAP for at least 4 hours a night for at least 5 nights a week (or a total of 20 hours a week) and this definition has been accepted by the American Academy of Sleep Medicine, Centers for Medicare & Medicaid Services, and almost all third-party payers in the United States. Because normal sleep time is about 49 hours a week, the current definition of compliant therapy represents the use of PAP for 41% of normal sleep hours (20/49 = 41%). Published studies on PAP have shown that only 58% to 80% of patients accept PAP therapy,[9–11] and that 49% of patients are compliant in the first month of therapy.[8] The largest study to date, the Apnea Positive Pressure Long-term Efficacy Study (APPLES) was a 6-month, randomized, double-blind, 2-arm, sham-controlled, multicenter trial on a total of 1516 enrolled subjects. In this study, Kushida and colleagues[12] found when analyzing CPAP use over the prior month that the compliance rate at 6 months was only 39% in the active CPAP group. In addition, there are many patients who prefer other therapy besides PAP because of the social issues related to PAP use. PAP therapy options include continuous PAP (CPAP), bilevel positive airway pressure, and autoadjusting positive airway pressure. Adherence to therapy is similar with the various PAP modalities.

Patients cite several issues with PAP, including discomfort and inability to sleep while connected to an air pressure device. Heated and humidified air and adequate education improve patient compliance, but compliance rates remain low. Nasal obstruction is a common limitation to effective PAP use. Medical treatments for nasal obstruction are typically tried first but, when not effective, nasal surgery may be indicated.

In the medical literature, a surgical cure is generally defined as a greater than 50% reduction in AHI and a final AHI of less than 20/h, but any reduction in AHI represents a reduction of disease burden and, in theory, should result in an overall improvement in morbidity and mortality.

## THE ROLE OF THE NOSE AND NASAL OBSTRUCTION IN OBSTRUCTIVE SLEEP APNEA

Nasal obstruction is a common complaint in patients with sleep disordered breathing, occurring in up to 45% of patients.[13,14] Nasal airway resistance is responsible for approximately two-thirds of total airway resistance. Increasing nasal resistance and nasal obstruction may be caused by a deviated septum, turbinate hypertrophy, internal or external nasal valve collapse, nasal mucosal inflammation, or space-occupying lesions in the nose (**Table 1**). Airway resistance is proportional to the length of the airway and inversely proportional to the fourth power of the radius.[15] As a result, a very small change in the size of the nasal airway caused by a septal spur, turbinate enlargement, internal or external nasal valve collapse, nasal polyp, or diffuse

| Table 1 | |
|---|---|
| **Causes of nasal obstruction** | |
| **Structural Problems** | **Mucosal/Inflammatory Problems** |
| Deviated septum | Allergic rhinitis |
| Nasal deformities/injuries | Nonallergic (vasomotor) rhinitis |
| Inferior turbinate hypertrophy | Rhinitis of pregnancy |
| Middle turbinate concha bullosa | Rhinitis medicamentosa |
| Nasal polyps | Wegener granulomatosis |
| Inverting papilloma | Sarcoidosis |
| Neoplasm | Medications (eg, β-blockers, estrogens) |
| Septal perforation | Atrophic rhinitis |
| Nasal synechia | Viral rhinitis |
| Nasal valve collapse | Bacterial rhinosinusitis |
| Choanal atresia | Fungal rhinosinusitis |
| Pyriform aperture stenosis | Tobacco use |
| Adenoid hypertrophy | |
| Nasopharyngeal cysts/tumors | |
| Meningocele/encephalocele | |
| Foreign body | |

inflammation can cause a very large increase in nasal airway resistance. The anterior nasal cavity has more effect on nasal airway resistance than the posterior nasal cavity because the smallest part of the airway is located anteriorly at the level of the internal nasal valve.

Nasal obstruction may cause or exacerbate sleep disordered breathing in many ways, including increasing upper airway resistance, causing sleep onset and sleep maintenance insomnia, worsening sleep fragmentation, increased work of breathing, and causing mouth breathing. In addition, nasal obstruction may reduce the stimulation of nasal receptors, leading to a depressed central respiratory drive and worsening of the AHI.[16] Oral breathing is likely detrimental to sleep quality. Nasal breathing has been shown to improve minute ventilation and pharyngeal muscle activity, whereas oral breathing worsens it.[17] Nasal breathing is also worse at night because of a circadian variation in nasal resistance, possibly caused by a combination of reduced serum cortisol levels at night and changes in cytokine levels during sleep.[18] In addition, there is increased nasal mucosal and tissue congestion when sleeping because there are no valves in the veins of the head and neck and therefore venous pressure in the nose increases when recumbent.[19]

Several studies have investigated the effects of nasal obstruction on sleep in otherwise normal subjects. Lavie and colleagues[20] studied 10 normal young adults without any ear, nose, and throat abnormalities and found that partial and complete mechanical obstruction of the nasal passages led to a significant increase in the number of apneas during sleep, in the number of microarousals associated with nonapneic breathing, and in the amount of wake time during sleep. Other studies have found that nasal obstruction leads to increased apneas, hypopneas, arousals, awakenings, and sleep stage changes, and reduced delta sleep.[21–25] Multiple studies have found a greater prevalence of sleep disordered breathing in patients with nasal inflammation, such as allergic rhinitis. Young and colleagues[26] studied 911 patients with nasal congestion caused by allergic rhinitis, finding a higher risk of excessive daytime sleepiness, snoring, and nonrestorative sleep and a 1.8 times greater risk of having sleep disordered breathing. Several studies have shown that exacerbations of allergic rhinitis lead to an increase in sleep disordered breathing and disturbed sleep,[27,28] and other epidemiology studies have shown that nasal obstruction seems to be an independent risk factor for snoring and OSA.[29,30] Most importantly, increased nasal resistance has been associated with poor compliance with CPAP.[31]

Nasal packing after nasal surgery has been shown to have an adverse effect on sleep disordered breathing. Suratt and colleagues[32] studied 8 men with and without nasal packing and found an increase in the number of obstructive apneas and hypopneas per hour and, to a lesser extent, the number of minutes of central events per hour. Armengot and colleagues[33] evaluated 40 patients treated with nasal packing for epistaxis, finding that 92.5% showed poorer oxygen saturation and 47% had severe desaturation. Desaturation was greater in obese patients. Friedman and colleagues[34] studied 49 patients with sleep apnea who were undergoing nasal surgery. They did a sleep study on the first postoperative night with nasal packing in place and found that, compared with the preoperative sleep study, the RDI, snoring, and ODI worsened in patients with mild OSA but not in those with moderate or severe OSA. Similarly, Turhan and colleagues[35] studied 43 patients after septoplasty and compared the effects on polysomnographic measures of packing versus a transseptal suture, and found that the packing caused a greater increase in AHI and greater decrease in oxygen desaturation after surgery than in patients having no packing.

## NASAL SURGERY

Common nasal surgeries performed to improve nasal breathing and for sleep disordered breathing include septoplasty, turbinate reduction, and nasal valve reconstruction. Septoplasty involves straightening of the nasal septum. The procedure may be done under local or general anesthesia and a variety of techniques are used based on surgical training and type and position of the septal deviation. Reducing a few millimeters of anterior septal deviation has been shown to produce significant improvements in nasal airway resistance, whereas repair of a posterior septal deviation has a lesser effect on airway resistance.

Turbinate reduction involves a reduction in the size of the inferior or middle turbinates. The procedure may be done under local or general anesthesia and a variety of techniques are used. Techniques include partial resection, submucous resection, outfracture, surface cautery, submucosal cautery, laser treatment, radiofrequency treatment, and endoscopic excision of concha bullosa when a concha bullosa is present in the middle turbinate.

Nasal valve reconstruction involves reconstruction of the internal or external nasal valve. The procedure may be done under local or general anesthesia and a variety of techniques are used. These techniques include spreader grafts, ear cartilage Batten grafts, J flaps, and various intranasal and extranasal suture techniques. There is insufficient research on the individual surgeries to validate the efficacy of each procedure but all of them cause an increase in the nasal airway and reduced collapsibility of the nasal valves, and lead to a reduction in nasal airway resistance. It is likely than any nasal surgery that accomplishes these end points should have a similar effect on sleep apnea or CPAP compliance.

There are limited data on the effects of endoscopic sinus surgery on sleep apnea and it is not clear whether endoscopic sinus surgery alone has any direct impact on nasal airway resistance. However, when sinus surgery improves sinusitis, there is a secondary benefit of reducing inflammation in the nose, which improves nasal resistance.

## EFFECT OF MEDICAL TREATMENT OF NASAL OBSTRUCTION ON OBSTRUCTIVE SLEEP APNEA

Treatment of nasal obstruction with medication has been shown to be beneficial for sleep quality. An early report by Craig and colleagues[36] showed that, in a placebo-controlled study on patients with allergic rhinitis, nasal steroids improved sleep quality. Nasal steroid sprays have also been shown to be beneficial in the pediatric population with allergic rhinitis. One study found a reduction in AHI from 10.7 to 5.8/h following a long course of fluticasone nasal spray.[37] Other nasal medications likely have mixed effects on sleep apnea and sleep quality because of common side effects related to sedation and stimulation. Mechanical means to open the nasal airway have also been shown to be helpful for snoring and sleep apnea. Petruson[38] found that, when 10 patients used a nasal dilator, there was a significant decrease in snoring, and Hoijer and colleagues[39] found that a nasal dilator in 11 patients improved nasal airflow as measured by rhinomanometry while reducing the frequency and severity of OSA. The mean apnea index decreased by 47% from 18/h to 6.4/h and the minimum oxygen saturation improved from 78% to 84% along with a reduction in snoring as measured on sleep testing. In contrast, Hoffstein and colleagues[40] found that a nasal dilator reduced snoring intensity and snores per minute in delta sleep but not in any other sleep stage and had no effect on numbers of apneas, hypopneas, or oxygen saturation. In addition, in a double-blind, randomized controlled crossover study in 18 patients with upper airway resistance syndrome, Bahammam and colleagues[41] found that a nasal dilator reduced stage 1 sleep and overall desaturation time without reducing AHI.

## EFFECT OF SURGICAL TREATMENT OF NASAL OBSTRUCTION ON OBSTRUCTIVE SLEEP APNEA

Numerous publications have shown the benefit of septoplasty, turbinate reduction, and nasal valve repair on sleep disordered breathing. In 1983, Heimer and colleagues[42] reported on 3 patients who had a dramatic clinical improvement following septoplasty, along with a reduction in the number and duration of obstructive apneas on sleep testing. Fairbanks[43] questioned 113 patients who had nasal surgery for nasal obstruction about snoring, finding that 42% had snored before the surgery. Of that group, snoring was either eliminated or improved in 77%. Dayal and Phillipson[44] did nasal valve reconstruction on 6 patients with sleep disordered breathing and all had a subjective improvement in snoring and daytime somnolence, whereas 3 also had objective improvement in their sleep apnea.

More recent studies include a report by Schuaib and colleagues,[45] who reported on 26 consecutive adults with nasal obstruction who underwent functional septorhinoplasty. The mean AHI decreased from 24.7 to 16.0 (a 57% reduction; $P<.01$) and, when excluding those with BMI greater than 30 kg/m$^2$, the AHI decreased from 22.5 to 9.6. In a similar study, Moxness and Nordgard[46] found a significant reduction in AHI (from $17.4 \pm 14.4$/h to $11.7 \pm 8.2$/h; $P<.01$) following septoplasty and turbinate reduction. Ishii and colleagues[47] did a meta-analysis of the results of nasal surgery on OSA and pooled data from 10 studies on 320 patients, of which there were 2 randomized controlled studies, 7 prospective studies, and 1 retrospective study. The pooled data showed a significant improvement in both Epworth Sleepiness Scale and RDI but no significant change in AHI.[47]

In addition to nasal disorders causing nasal airway obstruction, it is well known that adenoid hypertrophy causes nasal obstruction. In addition, marked tonsil hypertrophy has been shown to increase nasal airway resistance and removal of the tonsils not only can improve sleep quality but can also improve nasal airway resistance.[48]

## EFFECT OF NASAL SURGERY ON OPTIMAL POSITIVE AIRWAY PRESSURE AND POSITIVE AIRWAY PRESSURE COMPLIANCE

It is generally thought that improving the nasal airway in patients with both nasal obstruction and poor PAP compliance should reduce the required PAP to control sleep apnea. Nonsurgical therapy to reduce nasal airway resistance has included the use of an internal nasal dilator, which reduced PAP requirement from 8.6 cwp (centimeters of water pressure) to 8.0 cwp in 38 patients undergoing testing with a CPAP autotitration device.[49] Because nasal surgery also improves the nasal resistance, nasal surgery on patients with nasal obstruction should also improve PAP adherence. Powell and colleagues[50] published the only prospective, randomized, double-blind, placebo-controlled trial on nasal surgery using temperature-controlled radiofrequency (TCRF) turbinate reduction on 22 patients with nasal obstruction interfering with use of CPAP who had failed prior medical therapy. Patients were randomized to TCRF or placebo sham TCRF. PAP compliance was measured with a covert monitor using an autotitration CPAP machine. There was a significant improvement of the nasal airway in the treatment group only (patient visual analogue scale [VAS], and blinded examiner VAS). Objective CPAP use, self-reported CPAP adherence, and subjective tolerance all improved in the treatment group but not in the placebo group.

Nakata and colleagues[31] reviewed the effect of nasal surgery on CPAP use in 12 patients with severe OSA syndrome and nasal obstruction, all intolerant to CPAP, who were evaluated prospectively and compared with a control group of 410 patients on CPAP with a mean airway resistance of 0.24 Pa/cm$^3$ as measured by rhinomanometry. Nasal surgery improved nasal airway resistance in all 12 patients from 0.57 Pa/cm$^3$ to 0.16 Pa/cm$^3$ ($P<.05$) and all 12 became tolerant to CPAP. In addition, the Epworth Sleepiness Scale in these patients improved from 11.7 to 3.3, LSAT improved from 68.3% to 75.3%, and CPAP optimal pressure decreased from 16.8 cwp to 12.0 cwp in 5 out of 12 who had obtained a preoperative optimal, but the AHI did not change following nasal surgery.

In a study on the effects of various nasal surgeries on CPAP use, Zonato and colleagues[51] did a retrospective study of 17 patients (of whom 3 also had tonsillectomy) with severe OSA (mean AHI, 38/h) who were unable to tolerate CPAP. CPAP optimal pressure was reduced from 12.4 cwp to 10.2 cwp ($P<.001$). Optimal CPAP was reduced more than 1 cwp in 76% and greater than or equal to 3 cwp in 41%.

Other investigators reported the effects of nasal surgery on CPAPs and compliance in case series reports. The series reported on 7 patients intolerant to CPAP who underwent nasal surgery and all improved their CPAP compliance and reduced the pressure required.[52] Similarly, Friedman and colleagues[53] reported on 50 patients who underwent nasal surgery for OSA and found that 49 of the 50 (98%) had improved nasal breathing, snoring improved or was gone in 17 (34%), excessive daytime sleepiness improved in 78%, the optimal CPAP was reduced ($P<.01$), but RDI and LSAT did not change.

In the largest evaluation to date of nasal surgery on CPAP use, Camacho and colleagues[54] did a meta-analysis of all published articles on nasal surgery and their effect on CPAP requirements and use. They found a total of 36 articles on the subject and analyzed 18 that met criteria for review, of which all but 1 was a retrospective or prospective case series. Seven studies (82 patients) were analyzed regarding therapeutic CPAP, finding that optimal pressure was reduced following nasal surgery from a mean of 11.6 ± 2.2 cwp to 9.5 ± 2.0 cwp with a mean difference (MD) of −2.66 cwp

(P<.00001). Further analysis was done on those studies that used only a nasal mask interface (nasal pillows could skew results because the pillow opens the nasal valve area). Of the remaining 5 studies using only the nasal masks (49 patients), the optimal nasal CPAP reduced from a mean of 11.3 ± 2.0 cwp to 8.8 ± 1.9 cwp with an MD of −2.81 cwp (P<.00001).

In the same study, Camacho and colleagues[54] analyzed the type of nasal surgery in a subgroup of 4 publications. The largest MD in CPAP occurred in the septoplasty and turbinate reduction group (25 patients) with an MD of −2.6 cwp (P<.00001) and less improvement following other nasal surgeries: unspecified (48 patients) with MD of −1.90 cwp (P = .0001), turbinate reduction only (8 patients) with an MD of −2.2 cwp (P = .048), and septoplasty only (1 patient) with an MD of −2.0 cwp.

Camacho and colleagues[54] also analyzed 11 publications (153 patients) for CPAP compliance (although terminology included compliance, adherence, tolerance, acceptance, or use) before and after nasal surgery, finding 3 studies with objective reports, 3 with subjective patient reports, and 6 that did not specify how the data were obtained. Regular use of CPAP before nasal surgery was 38.7% (36 of 93 patients) improving to 90.2% (92 of 102 patients) after surgery. In addition, 89.1% (57 of 64 patients) who were unable to use CPAP before surgery were able to used it afterward. In the objective studies, the mean use of CPAP was 3.0 ± 3.1 hours and 5.5 ± 2.0 hours before and after surgery.

## REFERENCES

1. Young T, Palta M, Dempsey J, et al. The occurrence of sleep-disordered breathing in middle-aged adults. N Engl J Med 1993;328:1230–5.
2. Fletcher EC, DeBehnke RD, Lovoi MS, et al. Undiagnosed sleep apnea in patients with essential hypertension. Ann Intern Med 1985;103:190–5.
3. Millman RP, Redline S, Carlisle CC, et al. Daytime hypertension in obstructive sleep apnea: prevalence and contributing risk factors. Chest 1991;99:861–6.
4. Partinen M, Palomaki H. Snoring and cerebral infarction. Lancet 1985;2:1325–6.
5. Koskenvuo M, Kaprio J, Telakivi T, et al. Snoring as a risk factor for ischaemic heart disease and stroke in men. BMJ 1987;294:16–9.
6. Hung J, Whitford EG, Parsons RW, et al. Association of sleep apnoea with myocardial infarction in men. Lancet 1990;336:261–4.
7. Malone S, Liu PP, Holloway R, et al. Obstructive sleep apnoea in patients with dilated cardiomyopathy: effects of continuous positive airway pressure. Lancet 1991;338:1480–4.
8. Kribbs NB, Pack AI, Kline LR, et al. Objective measurement of patterns of nasal CPAP use by patients with obstructive sleep apnea. Am Rev Respir Dis 1993; 147(4):887–95.
9. Waldhorn RE, Herrick TW, Nguyen MC, et al. Long-term compliance with nasal continuous positive airway pressure therapy of obstructive sleep apnea. Chest 1990;97:33–8.
10. Meurice JC, Dore P, Paquereau J, et al. Predictive factors of long term compliance with nasal continuous positive airway pressure treatment in sleep apnea syndrome. Chest 1994;105:429–33.
11. Rauscher H, Formanek D, Popp W, et al. Nasal CPAP and weight loss in hypertensive patients with obstructive sleep apnea. Thorax 1993;48:529–33.
12. Kushida CA, Nichols DA, Holmes TH, et al. Effects of continuous positive airway pressure on neurocognitive function in obstructive sleep apnea patients: the

Apnea Positive Pressure Long-term Efficacy Study (APPLES). Sleep 2012;35(12): 1593–602.

13. Brander PE, Soirinsuo M, Lohela P. Nasopharyngeal symptoms in patients with obstructive sleep apnea syndrome. Effect of nasal CPAP treatment. Respiration 1999;66:128–35.

14. Pepin JL, Leger P, Veale D, et al. Side effects of nasal continuous positive airway pressure in sleep apnea syndrome. study of 193 patients in two French sleep centers. Chest 1995;107:375–81.

15. Susarla SM, Thomas RJ, Abramson ZR, et al. Biomechanics of the upper airway: changing concepts in the pathogenesis of obstructive sleep apnea. Int J Oral Maxillofac Surg 2010;39:1149–59.

16. White D, Cadieux R, Lomard R, et al. The effects of nasal anesthesia on breathing during sleep. Am Rev Respir Dis 1985;132:972–5.

17. McNicholas W, Coffey M, Boyle T. Effects of nasal airflow on breathing during sleep in normal humans. Am Rev Respir Dis 1993;147:620–3.

18. Craig TJ, Ferguson BJ, Krouse JH. Sleep impairment in allergic rhinitis, rhinosinusitis and nasal polyposis. Am J Otol 2008;29:209–17.

19. Desfonds P, Planes C, Fuhrman C, et al. Nasal resistance in snorers with or without sleep apnea: effect of posture and nasal ventilation with continuous positive airway pressure. Sleep 1998;15(6):625–32.

20. Lavie P, Fischel J, Zomer J, et al. The effects of partial and complete mechanical occlusion of the nasal passages on sleep structure and breathing in sleep. Acta Otolaryngol 1983;95:161–6.

21. Zwillich C, Zimmerman J, Weil J. Effects of nasal obstruction on sleep in normal men. Clin Res 1979;27:405a.

22. Zwillich C, Pickett C, Hanson F, et al. Disturbed sleep and prolonged apnea during nasal obstruction in normal men. Am Rev Respir Dis 1981;124:158–60.

23. Olsen K, Kern E, Westbrook P. Sleep and breathing disturbance secondary to nasal obstruction. Otolaryngol Head Neck Surg 1981;89:804–10.

24. Wilhoit S, Suratt P. Effect of nasal obstruction on upper airway muscle activation in normal subjects. Chest 1987;92:1053–5.

25. Lavie P, Rubin E. Effects of nasal occlusion on respiration in sleep. Acta Otolaryngol 1984;97:127–30.

26. Young T, Finn L, Palta M. Chronic nasal congestion at night is a risk factor for snoring in population-based cohort study. Arch Intern Med 2001;161:1514–9.

27. Lavie P, Gertner R, Zomer J, et al. Breathing disorders in sleep associated with microarousals in patients with allergic rhinitis. Acta Otolaryngol 1981;92:529–33.

28. McNicholas W, Tarlo S, Cole P, et al. Obstructive apneas during sleep in patients with seasonal allergic rhinitis. Am Rev Respir Dis 1982;126:625–8.

29. Stradling JR, Crosby JH. Predictors and prevalence of obstructive sleep apnea in 1001 middle-aged men. Thorax 1991;46:85–90.

30. Lofaso F, Coste A, d'Ortho MP, et al. Nasal obstruction as a risk factor for sleep apnoea syndrome. Eur Respir J 2000;16:639–43.

31. Nakata S, Noda A, Yagi H, et al. Nasal resistance for determinant factor of nasal surgery in CPAP failure patients with obstructive sleep apnea syndrome. Rhinology 2005;43(4):296–9.

32. Suratt PM, Turner BL, Wilhoit SC. Effect of intranasal obstruction on breathing during sleep. Chest 1986;90(3):324–9.

33. Armengot M, Hernandez R, Miguel P, et al. Effect of total nasal obstruction on nocturnal oxygen saturation. Am J Rhinol 2008;22(3):325–8.

34. Friedman M, Maley A, Kelley K. Impact of nasal obstruction on obstructive sleep apnea. Otolaryngol Head Neck Surg 2011;144(6):1000–4.
35. Turhan M, Bostanci A, Akdag M, et al. A comparison of the effects of packing or transseptal suture on polysomnographic parameters in septoplasty. Eur Arch Otorhinolaryngol 2013;20(4):1339–44.
36. Craig T, Teets S, Lehman E, et al. Nasal congestion secondary to allergic rhinitis as a cause of sleep disturbance and daytime fatigue and the response to topical nasal corticosteroids. J Allergy Clin Immunol 1998;101:633–7.
37. Brouillette RT, Manoukian JJ, Ducharme FM, et al. Efficacy of fluticasone nasal spray for pediatric obstructive sleep apnea. J Pediatr 2001;138:838–44.
38. Petruson B. Snoring can be reduced when the nasal airflow is increased by the nasal dilator Nozovent. Arch Otolaryngol 1990;116:462–4.
39. Hoijer U, Ejnell H, Hedner J, et al. The effects of nasal dilation on snoring and obstructive sleep apnea. Arch Otolaryngol Head Neck Surg 1992;118:281–4.
40. Hoffstein V, Mateika S, Metes A. Effect of nasal dilation on snoring and apneas during different stages of sleep. Sleep 1993;16(4):360–5.
41. Bahammam AS, Tate R, Manfreda J, et al. Upper airway resistance syndrome: effect of nasal dilation, sleep stage, and sleep position. Sleep 1999;22:592–8.
42. Heimer D, Scharf SM, Lieberman A, et al. Sleep apnea syndrome treated by repair of deviated nasal septum. Chest 1983;84:184–5.
43. Fairbanks DNF. Effect of nasal surgery on snoring. South Med J 1985;78(3):268–70.
44. Dayal VS, Phillipson EA. Nasal surgery in the management of sleep apnea. Ann Otol Rhinol Laryngol 1985;94:550–4.
45. Schuaib SW, Undavia S, Lin J, et al. Can functional septorhinoplasty independently treat obstructive sleep apnea? Plast Reconstr Surg 2015;135(6):1554–65.
46. Moxness MH, Nordgard S. An observational cohort study of the effects of septoplasty with or without inferior turbinate reduction in patients with obstructive sleep apnea. BMC Ear Nose Throat Disord 2014;21(14):11.
47. Ishii L, Roxbury C, Godoy A, et al. Does nasal surgery improve OSA in patients with nasal obstruction and OSA? A meta-analysis. Otolaryngol Head Neck Surg 2015;153(3):326–33.
48. Nakata S, Miyazaki S, Ohki M, et al. Reduced nasal resistance after simple tonsillectomy in patients with OSA. Am J Rhinol 2007;21:192–5.
49. Schonhofer B, Kerl J, Suchi S, et al. Effect of nasal valve dilation on effective CPAP level in obstructive sleep apnea. Respir Med 2007;97:1001–5.
50. Powell NB, Zanato AI, Weaver EM, et al. Radiofrequency treatment of turbinate hypertrophy in subjects using continuous positive airway pressure: a randomized, double-blind, placebo-controlled clinical pilot trial. Laryngoscope 2001;111(10):1783–90.
51. Zonato AI, Bittencourt LR, Martinho FL, et al. Upper airway surgery: the effect on nasal continuous positive airway pressure titration on obstructive sleep apnea patients. Eur Arch Otorhinolaryngol 2006;263(5):481–6.
52. Series F, St Pierre S, Carrier G. Effects of surgical correction of nasal obstruction in the treatment of obstructive sleep apnea. Am Rev Respir Dis 1992;146:1261–5.
53. Friedman M, Tanyeri H, Lim JW, et al. Effect of improved nasal breathing on obstructive sleep apnea. Otolaryngol Head Neck Surg 2000;122:71–4.
54. Camacho M, Riaz M, Capasso R, et al. The effect of nasal surgery on continuous positive airway pressure device use and therapeutic treatment pressures: a systematic review and meta-analysis. Sleep 2015;38(2):279–86.

# Palatal Procedures for Obstructive Sleep Apnea

Kathleen Yaremchuk, MD, MSA

## KEYWORDS

- Uvulopalatopharyngoplasty • Laser-assisted uvulopalatoplasty
- Radiofrequency volumetric tissue reduction • Palatal implants
- Lateral pharyngoplasty • Cautery-assisted palatal stiffening operation
- Z palatoplasty

## KEY POINTS

- Uvulopalatoplasty is used to treat patients with obstructive sleep apnea (OSA) who have narrowing of the retro-palatal area of the pharynx.
- There have been many descriptions of procedures for the palate to decrease its length and move it anteriorly to increase the anterior posterior dimensions of the inferior margin of the palate.
- New techniques using radio frequency, laser, and implants have been used for snoring and OSA; but results have been similar to more surgically oriented techniques.

The procedure uvulopalatopharyngoplasty (UPPP) was first described for the treatment of snoring by Ikematsu in 1964.[1] Much later, in 1981, UPPP was described by Fujita and colleagues as "a new surgical approach" to treat obstructive sleep apnea.[2] Until then, permanent tracheostomy had been the only consistently effective surgical treatment in adult sleep apnea[3] but resulted in psychosocial issues that were unacceptable to many patients. Fujita and colleagues described 12 predominantly male (11 of 12) patients with a history of excessive daytime sleepiness and loud habitual snoring. The velopharyngeal space was identified as the area of functional collapse of the pharynx during apneas. Clinically, the patients had a shallow oropharyngeal space with a relatively large uvula and redundant mucosa of the surrounding tissue.[2]

Fujita and colleagues[4] subsequently described a series of 66 patients (63 men) treated for obstructive sleep apnea with UPPP. The mean apnea index (AI) preoperatively was 59. Significant improvements occurred after UPPP, although great variability was noted in individual patient response. Two subgroups were identified: responders (33 of 66) showed a significant decrease in AI of 84% (58.3–9.5), whereas

Disclosure Statement: The author has nothing to disclose.
Department of Otolaryngology/Head and Neck Surgery, Henry Ford Hospital, 2799 West Grand Boulevard, Detroit, MI 48202, USA
E-mail address: kyaremc1@hfhs.org

nonresponders had little improvement (60.3–55.4). Despite recognizing the clear variability in response, they were unable to identify a sleep or respiratory parameter that differentiated the response to UPPP.

Some explored whether patients with mild sleep apnea might be more likely to benefit from surgical treatment. In an evaluation of 37 unselected patients with mild obstructive sleep apnea who underwent UPPP, Senior and colleagues[5] found that only 40% had at least a 50% postoperative reduction in the respiratory event index (REI). Other patients had an increase in average REI from 161.6 ±5.0 to 26.7 ±18.4. Subjective assessment of sleepiness similarly was not improved. Again, the issue of responders and nonresponders arose.

In a review of the literature, Sher and colleagues[6] noted that reports of case series and few controlled trials tend to limit the ability to advocate for change in surgical practice across the specialty. Their review found that UPPP was effective, at best, in less than 50% of patients with obstructive sleep apnea.

The variability in results of UPPP and the inability to predict which patients would respond to surgery became frustrating to otolaryngologists as many sleep medicine physicians refrained from referring patients for surgical interventions. Because of a success rate that was quoted as a 50:50 chance of improvement, many otolaryngologists attempted to improve surgical success results and to decrease the postoperative period in patients with obstructive sleep apnea with modifications of the traditional UPPP.

A breakthrough began when Friedman and colleagues[7,8] classified patients with obstructive sleep apnea with a staging system based on body mass index (BMI), tonsil size, and palate position. Stage I was defined as a palate position 1 or 2 combined with tonsil size 3 or 4. Stage II was defined as palate position 3 or 4 and tonsil size 3 or 4. Stage III patients had palate position 3 or 4 and tonsil size 0, 1, or 2. Any patient with a BMI greater than 40 was stage III. In a retrospective analysis, UPPP alone had an 80% success rate in stage I patients, 37.9% success in stage II, and 8.1% success in stage III (**Fig. 1**, **Table 1**).

Multiple palatal procedures were developed to improve surgical success. An attempt to review all published procedures would be difficult because most are single series by individual surgeons and did not include large enough numbers or the technique was not adopted by others to reach significance within the specialty. Some of the procedures included new technology that was developed or applied in a novel way.

## UVULOPALATOPHARYNGOPLASTY

Fujita described the UPPP as a procedure to remove redundant mucosa and preserve the muscular layer to enlarge the oropharyngeal space.[2] The procedure required general anesthesia, and patients were admitted to the hospital. The UPPP was performed by making an incision through the mucosa of the soft palate lateral to the glossopalatal arch from the inferior pole of the tonsillar fossa toward the uvula ending at its tip. The incision was extended on the pharyngeal side of the uvula and the pharyngopalatal arch toward the inferior pole of the tonsil. The mucosa of the soft palate, tonsillar fossa, and the lateral aspect of the uvula were undermined with sharp dissection and excised. The mucosal edges between the anterior and postural palatal arches were reapproximated with interrupted sutures. This maneuver brought the palatal arch forward or anteriorly with an increase in the anterior posterior dimension of the oropharyngeal space. If the uvula was elongated with the maneuver, then it was shortened or removed. If redundant tissue was in the posterior pharyngeal wall, an additional

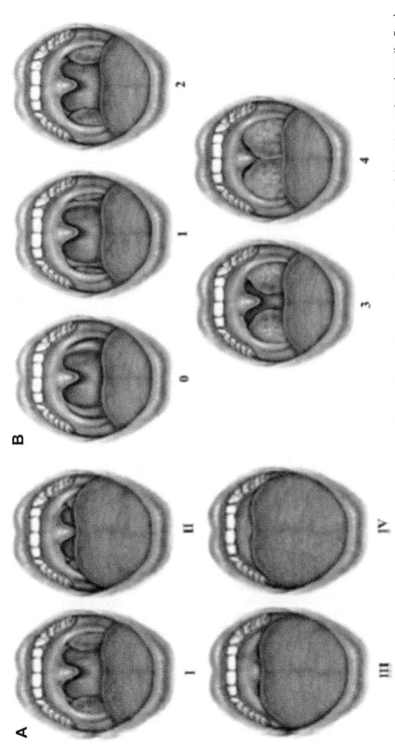

**Fig. 1.** (A) The Friedman palate position is based on visualization of the oral cavity. Palate grade I has visualization of the entire uvula and tonsils. Grade II has visualization of the uvula but not the tonsils. Grade III shows visualization of the soft palate, and grade IV reveals only the hard palate. (B) Tonsil size is graded from 0 to 4. Size 0 tonsils are surgically removed. Size 1 tonsils are tonsils hidden within the pillars. Size 2 tonsils are extending to the pillars. Size 3 tonsils are beyond the pillars but not the midline. Size 4 tonsils are touching in the midline. (*From* Friedman M, Ibrahim H, Bass L. Clinical staging for sleep disordered breathing. Otolaryngol Head Neck Surg 2002;127:14–5; with permission.)

**Table 1**
**Friedman staging system based on Friedman tongue position, tonsil size, and body mass index**

|           | Friedman Tongue Position | Tonsil Size | BMI |
|-----------|--------------------------|-------------|-----|
| Stage I   | 1                        | 3, 4        | <40 |
|           | 2                        | 3, 4        | <40 |
| Stage II  | 1, 2                     | 0, 1, 2     | <40 |
|           | 3, 4                     | 3, 4        | <40 |
| Stage III | 3, 4                     | 0, 1, 2     | <40 |
|           | Any                      | Any         | >40 |

*From* Friedman M, Ibrahim H, Bass L. Clinical staging for sleep disordered breathing. Otolaryngol Head Neck Surg 2002;127:16; with permission.

excision of the posterior pharyngeal mucosa could be done. The posterior pharyngeal mucosa was elevated and stretched laterally and sutured (**Fig. 2**).

## THE UVULOPALATAL FLAP

The uvulopalatal flap (UPF) was reported by Powell and colleagues[9] who used a technique to advance the uvula and distal palate by creating a flap of tissue that was reversed on itself and sutured close to the hard palate. The advancement flap started with the ventral surface of the soft palate, and the uvula had the mucosa removed and was sutured in place. An incision was made that also released the lateral aspects of the palate. Huntley's[10] drawings described the steps of the procedure very well (see **Fig. 2**).[10] Initially, local anesthetic with a vasoconstrictor was injected in the ventral surface of the soft palate and uvula to assist with separating a plane between the muscular layer and the mucosa, which also helped with pain control and hemostasis. The soft palate and uvula were retracted toward the hard palate to allow an outline to be drawn for the incision. The ventral mucosa was removed, and relaxing incisions were made at the lateral aspect to provide greater anterior release of the UPF and increase the retro-palatal area. The palate was then folded on itself, and the mucosa of the dorsal palate and uvula was sutured into position.

The procedure can be done as an outpatient or under general anesthesia. An advantage was that the procedure was potentially reversible if velopharyngeal insufficiency occurred. Because muscular tissue was not removed, the normal physiologic mobility of the palate was maintained and the likelihood of scar contracture and subsequent nasopharyngeal stenosis would be decreased. An important additional benefit was a decrease in postoperative pain because there was no disruption of muscle tissue or presence of denuded surfaces.

An extended UPF (EUPF) described by Li and colleagues[11] included the previous procedure but used dissection and removal of submucosal adipose tissue of the soft palate and supratonsillar area (**Fig. 3**). The EUPF was done in conjunction with tonsillectomy. The EUPF was done under general anesthesia, and in their series there was one occurrence of bleeding from the tonsillar fossa during the postoperative period and 3% of patients had occasional nasal regurgitation.

Surgical success was reported in 81.8% based on a 50% or greater decrease and less than 20 apnea-hypopnea index (AHI) reported in 27 men with only retro-palatal obstruction. The mean BMI in this series was 26.7, which is less than usual patients with obstructive sleep apnea in the United States but was considered "overweight for middle aged Taiwanese."

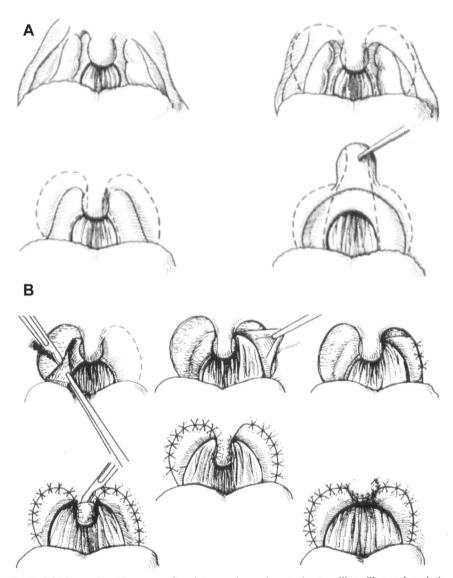

**Fig. 2.** (*A*) Mucosal incisions on soft palate, uvula, and posterior tonsillar pillar and uvula in UPPP. (*B*) Excision of redundant mucosa from the soft palate, uvula, and posterior pillar and reapproximation of tissue. (*From* Fujita S, Conway W, Zorick F, et al. Surgical correction of anatomic abnormalities in obstructive sleep apnea syndrome: uvulopalatopharyngoplasty. Otolaryngol Head Neck Surg 1981;89:926–27; with permission.)

## LASER-ASSISTED UVULOPALATOPHARYNGOPLASTY

Laser-assisted uvulopalatoplasty (LAUP) was described by Kamami[12] initially for the treatment of snoring and subsequently for the treatment of obstructive sleep apnea and as an alternative to UPPP.[12] The procedure was performed with the application of topical 10% lidocaine spray applied to the soft palate and base of tongue. Several milliliters of 1% lidocaine with 1:100,000 epinephrine was then injected into the soft

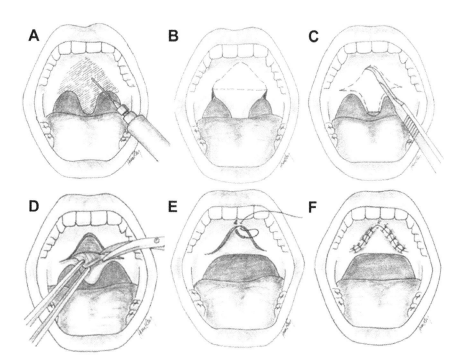

**Fig. 3.** (A) Local anesthetic with vasoconstrictive agent is injected in the shaded area after application of topic anesthetic. (B) In the case of excessive tonsillar pillar webbing or a long soft palate, additional advancement of the tissue can be obtained by placement of re-laxing incisions that extend superiorly. (C) Mucosal incisions are performed with lateral extension. The distal uvula may require shortening. (D) The mucosa is undermined and removed with sharp dissection and cautery used for hemostasis. (E) Closure being at the central aspect of the flap with a mattress suture. (F) Interrupted sutures complete the closure. (*From* Huntley T. The uvulopalatal flap. Operat Tech Otolaryngol Head Neck Surg 2000;11(1):31–3; with permission.)

palate. Appropriate laser precautions (protective eye wear, smoke evacuator) were used. The laser was set at 15 to 20 W, and a handpiece with a backstop designed to protect the posterior pharyngeal wall was used to make a vertical incision 1.0 to 1.5 cm on each side of the uvula through the soft palate. This procedure was followed by partial vaporization of the free edge of the uvula and possibly the lateral aspects of the soft palate to shorten the length.

Hemostasis could be controlled with silver nitrate or other topical agents. Patients were sent home with pain medications and possibly antibiotics. LAUPs were sometimes staged so that if residual symptoms were present, then a subsequent procedure could be performed. A concern was that with healing and contracture of the burned tissue, velopharyngeal insufficiency could occur. Walker[13] and Mickelson[14] reported surgical success as defined as a decrease of 50% AHI in 47.4% and 53.8% of patients with retro-palatal obstruction treated with LAUP.

Finkelstein and colleagues[15] evaluated 174 patients with heavy snoring or obstructive sleep apnea and compared UPPP with LAUP. The first 100 consecutive patients underwent conventional UPPP, and the subsequent 74 had LAUP performed. Sleep parameters were not measured before or after the procedure; however, anatomic measurements noted circumferential scarring in the LAUP patients, resulting in medial retraction and reduction in circumferential space at the level of the palate. This result could have been secondary to technique or excessive heat causing collateral damage to adjacent tissue.

Much of LAUP's appeal was its ability to be performed on an outpatient basis with topical and local anesthetic. It was described as cost-effective because it avoided the cost of the operating room and subsequent hospitalization. The expense of a laser, however, was cost prohibitive for many practitioners.

## CAUTERY-ASSISTED PALATAL STIFFENING OPERATION

Cautery-assisted palatal stiffening operation (CAPSO) was an outpatient procedure used for snoring and sleep apnea. Of 25 consecutive patients with obstructive sleep apnea who underwent CAPSO, responders were defined as patients with a 50% or more reduction and less than 10 AHI. With these strict criteria, 40% of patients demonstrated success.[16] For treatment of habitual snoring, 206 patients were treated; a success rate of 92% was found initially, which decreased to 77% after a year.[17]

The procedure was performed with topical anesthetic applied and then 5 mL of 2% lidocaine with 1:100,000 epinephrine injected into the midline soft palate. A blended cautery with needle tip was used to outline an inverted U on the soft palate. A 2-cm piece of mucosa was removed in a superior to inferior direction. The denuded tissue was cauterized to further stiffen the tissue and for hemostasis. The wound was allowed to heal by secondary intention (**Fig. 4**).

## LATERAL PHARYNGOPLASTY

Many surgeons had noted that the traditional UPPP may fail because of lateral pharyngeal wall collapse. Cahali described lateral pharyngoplasty, a new surgical technique designed to splint lateral pharyngeal wall collapse.[18] In a prospective, randomized study, 27 patients were randomly assigned to UPPP or lateral pharyngoplasty.[19] Lateral pharyngoplasty showed a greater decrease in the AHI than in the UPPP group ($P = .05$).

The procedure was performed under general anesthesia with a McIvor mouth gag in place to give adequate exposure. A tonsillectomy was performed or the tonsillar fossa mucosa was removed to identify the palatoglossus and palatopharyngeus muscles. With the use of a microscope, the superior pharyngeal constrictor (SPC) muscle was undermined and elevated. The SPC muscle was sectioned caudally resulting in muscle flaps that were sutured anteriorly to the same-side palatoglossus muscle (**Fig. 5**). An incision was made from the lateral base of the uvula extending diagonally laterally of the upper part of the palatopharyngeus muscle, which created a palatine laterally based flap. A transverse subtotal section of the palatopharyngeus muscle was made in its superior part creating a superior and an inferior flap. The superior and palatine flaps were sutured in a z-plasty fashion. The anterior to the posterior tonsillar pillars were sutured. Then the distal third of the uvula was removed.

## EXPANSION SPHINCTER PHARYNGOPLASTY

Expansion sphincter pharyngoplasty (ESP) was described by Pang and Woodson[20] to prevent lateral wall collapse in patients with obstructive sleep apnea.[20] In a prospective, randomized controlled trial, 45 adults with a BMI less than 30, Friedman stage II or III, and with lateral wall collapse had either traditional UPPP or the ESP. Using a surgical success definition of a 50% reduction and less than 20 AHI, ESP had 82.6% success compared with 68.1% in UPPP ($P<.05$).

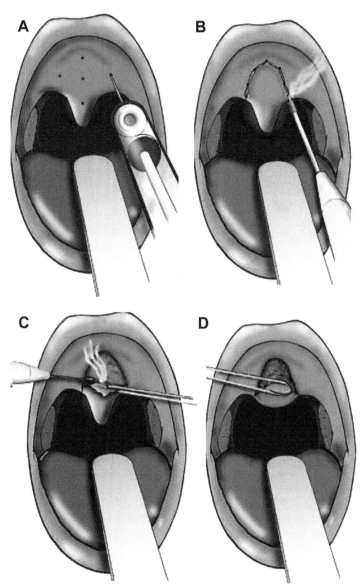

**Fig. 4.** (*A*) Topical anesthetic with vasoconstrictive agent is injected into the soft palate. (*B*) Electrocautery is used to outline the area of elevation. Cautery and forceps are used to elevate the mucosal soft palatal flap 1 cm from the junction of the hard and soft palate to the tip of the uvula. (*C*) An inverted U incision is made dissecting the mucosa off of the uvular ridge. Cauterization of the midline mucosa on the nasopharyngeal surface of the uvula enhances the stiffening effect. (*D*) The specimen is removed, and the central palatal musculature remains intact. (*From* Mair E, Day R. Cautery-assisted palatal stiffening operation. Otolaryngol Head Neck Surg 2000;122(4):548; with permission.)

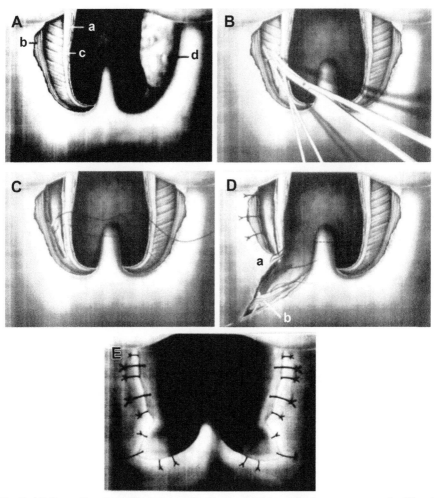

**Fig. 5.** (*A*) Operative view after left tonsillectomy with (a) palatopharyngeus muscle, (b) palatoglossus muscle, (c) superior pharyngeal constrictor muscle, and (d) right tonsil. (*B*) Elevation and section of the left superior pharyngeal constrictor muscle. (*C*) Anterior suture of the superior pharyngeal constrictor muscle (lateral flap) to the palatoglossus muscle. (*D*) Z-plasty covering the superior part of the tonsillar fossa: (a) palatine flap, (b) upper part of the palatopharyngeus muscle. Incision to remove part of the uvula (*dashed line*). (*E*) Final aspect of the lateral pharyngoplasty. (*From* Cahali M. Lateral pharyngoplasty: a new treatment for obstructive sleep apnea hypopnea syndrome. Laryngoscope 2003;113:1962–64; with permission.)

The procedure was performed under general anesthesia. A tonsillectomy was performed, and the palatopharyngeus muscle was identified and the inferior end transected and rotated superolaterally. The muscle was left with its posterior surface partially attached to the horizontal superior pharyngeal constrictor muscles. Enough muscle had to be isolated to allow suturing. An incision was made on the anterior pillar identifying the palatoglossus muscles. The palatopharyngeus muscle was then attached to the arching fibers of the soft palate. A partial uvulectomy was then performed and the incisions closed (**Fig. 6**).

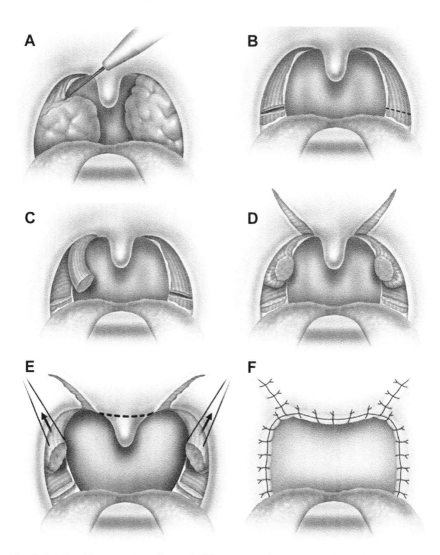

**Fig. 6.** (*A*) Tonsillectomy is performed. (*B*) Horizontal incision made to divide the inferior end of the palatopharyngeus muscle. (*C*) The palatopharyngeus muscle is mobilized, although not completely, with care taken to leave its fascia attachments to the deeper horizontal constrictor muscles. (*D*) Superolateral incision made on the soft palate, revealing the arching fibers of the palatine muscles. (*E*) Sutures are used to hitch up (*arrows*) the palatopharyngeus muscle to the soft palate muscles superolaterally. (*F*) Closure of the palatal incisions. (*From* Pang K, Woodson BT. Expansion sphincter pharyngoplasty: a new technique for the treatment of obstructive sleep apnea. Otolaryngol Head Neck Surg 2007;137:111–2; with permission.)

## Z-PALATOPLASTY

Friedman and colleagues[21] described a modification of uvulopalatopharyngoplasty based on a bilateral z-plasty in treating patients without tonsils and an unfavorable tongue position (Friedman tongue position [FTP] III and IV).[21] Patients who have had tonsillectomy often have posterior displacement of the palate. This displacement is thought to occur when the posterior tonsillar pillars have been resected and there is tissue contracture. The goal of the z-plasty is to increase the space between the palate and the postpharyngeal wall and between the palate and tongue base. This technique is thought to change the scar contracture tension line to an anterolateral direction and widens the anteroposterior and lateral oropharyngeal airway at the level of the palate.

Twenty-five patients treated with Z-palatoplasty (ZPP) were matched with 25 patients treated with classic UPPP. All patients in both groups were treated with radiofrequency tongue base reduction (TBRF), due to unfavorable FTP. Perioperative complications were rare in both groups. Temporary velopharyngeal insufficiency (VPI) was reported in the 12 ZPP and 7 UPPP patients. In all patients the VPI completely resolved by 3 months after surgery. No cases of permanent VPI were encountered in either group.

Objective measures of surgical success were AHI and the minimum recorded arterial oxygen saturation as recorded with polysomnography. Using a 50% or greater reduction in postoperative AHI and an AHI less than 20 the ZPP with TBRF resulted in a 68% success where the traditional UPP combined with TBRF had a 28% success rate.

The procedure is performed under general anesthesia. Two adjacent flaps are outlined on the palate. The mucosa of the anterior aspect of the two flaps is removed. The palatal segment splits the uvula and the inferior one-third to one-half of the soft palate in half. A 2-layer closure bringing the midline superior to the margin of the soft palate is performed. The lateral flaps are sewn laterally to the defect (**Fig. 7**).

## RADIOFREQUENCY VOLUMETRIC TISSUE REDUCTION

Radiofrequency volumetric tissue reduction (RVTR) for treatment of sleep-disordered breathing (SDB) was described by Powell and colleagues[22] in 1998. Radiofrequency ablation of soft tissue was used in the palate. This prospective, nonrandomized study of 22 healthy patients with mild SDB (AHI <15) and excessive daytime sleepiness reported improvements in sleep efficiency index ($P = .002$), subjective snoring scores (decrease by 77%), and mean Epworth sleepiness scores (8.5 ±4.4–5.2 ±3.3, $P = .0001$).

A subsequent prospective, nonrandomized study on 30 patients compared RVTR with LAUP for treatment of snoring. Patients with simple snoring or mild sleep apnea were included. Both treatments were effective in eliminating snoring, but the RVTR was better tolerated.[23]

A prospective clinical trial compared RVTR and UPPP in 79 consecutive patients. Preoperatively, the two groups had no difference of subjective symptoms, age, and BMI. The snoring scores improved significantly in both groups ($P<.001$). AHI showed significant improvement postoperatively in the UPPP group ($P = .025$) but not after RVTR.[24]

During this outpatient procedure in the clinic, the patients had topical application of lidocaine spray to the soft palate. The soft palate was then infiltrated with 2 to 3 mL of 2% lidocaine with 1:100,000 epinephrine in the midline and an additional 1.0 to 1.5 mL lateral to midline on each side. A bipolar radiofrequency electrode was placed in the submucosal layer of the soft palate in 3 different sites: the first in the midline vertically, then paramedian left, and right in a diagonal medial to lateral direction. Up to 3 treatments can be performed with a 6-week period of healing between treatments. Postoperative pain was managed with oral pain medication (**Fig. 8**).

## PILLAR PALATAL IMPLANTS

Pillar palatal implants, or polyethylene terephthalate implants, when inserted in the soft palate cause an inflammatory reaction that leads to the formation of a fibrous

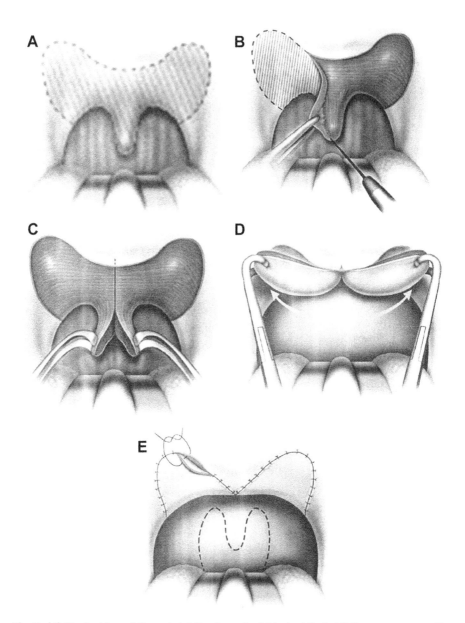

**Fig. 7.** (*A*) The incision of the palatal flap is marked (*dashed line*). (*B*) The mucosa over the palatal flap is removed, exposing the palatal musculature. (*C*) The uvula and palate are split in the midline with a scalpel. (*D*) The uvular flaps are reflected posteriorly and laterally over the soft palate (*arrows*). (*E*) A 2-layered closure of the palatal flaps is performed. (*From* Friedman M, Ibrahim H, Vidyasagar R, et al. Z-palatoplasty (ZPP): a technique for patients without tonsils. Otolaryngol Head Neck Surg 2004;131(1):91–5; with permission.)

encapsulation of the implants. The fibrosis that occurs stiffens the soft palate and decreases palatal fluttering. The increased rigidity decreases the AHI. The pillar palatal implants were performed as an outpatient procedure with little pain or discomfort, an attractive alternative for some patients with snoring and sleep apnea.

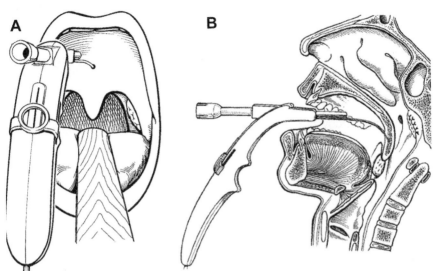

**Fig. 8.** (A) Radiofrequency treatment shows placement of the handpiece after local anesthetic is injected. (B) Lateral view of treatment procedure depicting placement of the electrode tip into the submucosal soft palate. The palate creates a lesion that is within the submucosal rather than mucosal tissue. (*From* Coleman, S, Smith T. Midline radiofrequency tissue reduction of the palate for bothersome snoring and sleep-disordered breathing; a clinical trial. Otolaryngol Head Neck Surg 2000;122:388; with permission.)

Friedman and colleagues[25] performed a prospective randomized study whereby patients received implants or a placebo. The pillar palatal treatment group's AHI significantly improved compared with the placebo group (7.9 ±7.7 vs 0.9 ±4.3). A different study randomized 100 patients to palatal implants or placebo. A success rate measured by a 50% decrease and less than 20 AHI occurred in the implant group compared with the sham group (26% vs 10%, $P = .05$).[26] Both studies were performed with 3 implants, but the manufacturer currently recommends the use of 5 implants for treatment.

The implants were done in the outpatient clinic setting. After rinsing the mouth with antiseptic oral rinse, local anesthetic was injected into the soft palate in the midline and adjacent left and right areas. Three pillar palate implants were injected, using the supplied handpiece, in the midline at the junction of the hard palate and soft palate and the paramedian left and right positions in a parallel manner.

## VARIATION ON A THEME

In reviewing the literature for this article, some articles on modified uvulopalatopharyngoplasty can best be described as variations on a theme; there were more than could be included in this article. Terms such as *EUPF, lateral inversion flap, snare uvulopalatoplasty*, and *resection of the musculus uvulae*, to name just a few, were procedures that were published for the treatment of obstructive sleep apnea.

On behalf of the American Academy of Sleep Medicine Standards of Practice, Caples and colleagues[27] conducted a systematic review and meta-analysis of the literature reporting outcomes for surgical treatment of obstructive sleep apnea. This review led to the conclusion that "most of the data are drawn from small case series of selected patients, in whom there were varied preoperative and surgical approaches. There were few controlled trials and varying approaches to pre-operative and post-operative follow up with inconsistent decreases in AHI."[27]

The uneven response to surgery, brings us back to the conundrum of responders and nonresponders[2] for patients with obstructive sleep apnea. For individuals with anatomic obstruction at the level of the tonsils or retropalatal areas, UPPP and tonsillectomy is successful in 80% of patients. When UPPP with or without tonsillectomy is done in unselected series of patients, the success rate decreases to 50% or lower.

## REFERENCES

1. Ikematsu T. Study of snoring, 4th report. J Jap Oto-Rhino-Laryngol 1964;64: 434–5.
2. Fujita S, Conway W, Zorick F, et al. Surgical correction of anatomic abnormalities in obstructive sleep apnea syndrome: uvulopalatopharyngoplasty. Otolaryngol Head Neck Surg 1981;89:923–34.
3. Conway W, Victor L, Magilligan D. Adverse effects of tracheostomy for obstructive sleep apnea. JAMA 1981;246:347–50.
4. Fujita S, Conway W, Zorick F, et al. Evaluation of the effectiveness of uvulopalatopharyngoplasty. Laryngoscope 1985;95:70–4.
5. Senior B, Rosenthal L, Lumley L, et al. Efficacy of uvulopalatopharyngoplasty in unselected patients with mild obstructive sleep apnea syndrome. Otolaryngol Head Neck Surg 2000;123:179–82.
6. Sher A, Schechtman K, Piccirrillo J. The efficacy of surgical modifications of the upper airway in patients with obstructive sleep apnea syndrome. Sleep 1996; 19(2):156–77.
7. Friedman M, Ibrahim H, Bass L. Clinical staging for sleep disordered breathing. Otolaryngol Head Neck Surg 2002;127:13–21.
8. Friedman M, Ibrahim H, Joseph N. Staging of obstructive sleep apnea/hypopnea syndrome: a guide to appropriate treatment. Laryngoscope 2004;114(3):454–9.
9. Powell N, Riley R, Guilleminault C, et al. A reversible uvulopalatal flap for snoring and sleep apnea syndrome. Sleep 1996;19:593–9.
10. Huntley T. The uvulopalatal flap. Operat Tech Otolaryngol Head Neck Surg 2000; 11(1):30–5.
11. Li H, Li K, Chen N, et al. Modified uvulopalatopharyngoplasty: the extended uvulopalatal flap. Am J Otolaryngol 2003;24(5):311–6.
12. Kamami YV. Outpatient treatment of sleep apnea syndrome with $CO_2$ laser, LAUP, laser-assisted UPPP results on 46 patients. J Clin Laser Med Surg 1994;12:215–9.
13. Walker R. Uvulopalatopharyngoplasty versus laser-assisted uvulopalatoplasty for the treatment of obstructive sleep apnea. Laryngoscope 1997;107(1):76–82.
14. Mickelson S. Laser-assisted uvulopalatoplasty for obstructive sleep apnea. Laryngoscope 1996;106(1):10–3.
15. Finkelstein Y, Shapiro-Feinberg M, Stein G, et al. Uvulopalatopharyngoplasty vs laser-assisted uvulopalatoplasty. Anatomical considerations. Arch Otolaryngol Head Neck Surg 1997;123:265–76.
16. Wassermuth Z, Mair E, Loube D, et al. Cautery-assisted palatal stiffening operation for the treatment of obstructive sleep apnea syndrome. Otolaryngol Head Neck Surg 2000;123(1):55–60.
17. Mair E, Day R. Cautery-assisted palatal stiffening operation. Otolaryngol Head Neck Surg 2000;122(4):547–56.
18. Cahali M. Lateral pharyngoplasty: a new treatment for obstructive sleep apnea hypopnea syndrome. Laryngoscope 2003;113:1961–8.

19. Cahali M, Formigoni G, Gebrim E, et al. Lateral pharyngoplasty versus uvulopalatopharyngoplasty: a clinical, polysomnographic and computer tomography measurement comparison. Sleep 2004;27(5):942–50.
20. Pang K, Woodson BT. Expansion sphincter pharyngoplasty: a new technique for the treatment of obstructive sleep apnea. Otolaryngol Head Neck Surg 2007;137: 110–4.
21. Friedman M, Ibrahim H, Vidyasagar R, et al. Z-palatoplasty (ZPP): a technique for patients without tonsils. Otolaryngol Head Neck Surg 2004;131(1):89–100.
22. Powell N, Riley R, Troell R, et al. Radiofrequency volumetric tissue reduction of the palate in subjects with sleep-disordered breathing. Chest 1998;113:1163–74.
23. Hofmann T, Schwantzer G, Reckenzaun E, et al. Radiofrequency tissue volume reduction of the soft palate and UPPP in the treatment of snoring. Eur Arch Otorhinolaryngol 2006;263:164–70.
24. Blumen M, Dahan S, Wagner I, et al. Radiofrequency versus LAUP for the treatment of snoring. Otolaryngol Head Neck Surg 2002;126(1):67–73.
25. Friedman M, Schlalch P, Lin H, et al. Palatal implants for the treatment of snoring and obstructive sleep apnea/hypopnea syndrome. Otolaryngol Head Neck Surg 2008;138:209–16.
26. Steward D, Huntley T, Woodson BT, et al. Palate implants or obstructive sleep apnea: multi-institution, randomized, placebo-controlled study. Otolaryngol Head Neck Surg 2008;139(4):506–10.
27. Caples S, Rowley J, Prinsell J, et al. Surgical modifications of the upper airway for obstructive sleep apnea in adults: a systematic review and meta-analysis. Sleep 2010;33(10):1396–407.

# Genioglossal Advancement, Hyoid Suspension, Tongue Base Radiofrequency, and Endoscopic Partial Midline Glossectomy for Obstructive Sleep Apnea

Jeffrey Dorrity, MD[a],*, Nicholas Wirtz, MD[a],
Oleg Froymovich, MD[b], David Hamlar, MD, DDS[a]

## KEYWORDS

- OSA • Radiofrequency • Tongue base • Hyoid suspension • Hyoid myotomy
- Genioglossus advancement • Sleep surgery • Genioplasty

## KEY POINTS

- Genioglossal advancement is designed for patients with collapse of the lower pharyngeal airway. With careful patient selection, it remains a viable option in the surgical management of OSA.
- Hyoid suspension has been shown to be an effective adjuvant to other sleep surgical procedures in a multistep surgical approach to OSA.
- Various techniques of volumetric reduction of the tongue have been supported by the literature for their positive impact in the reduction of the apnea-hypopnea index and relatively minimal operative morbidity and long-term complications.

## GENIOGLOSSUS ADVANCEMENT FOR TREATMENT OF OBSTRUCTIVE SLEEP APNEA

Surgical intervention for obstructive sleep apnea (OSA) is a complex topic. The discussion involves intricate procedures targeting specific areas of the upper airway. Because of the wide variety of physiologic and anatomic causes of this disorder it is important to tailor the treatment to offer the patient the best possible outcome. Fujita

Disclosures: N. Wirtz and D. Hamlar have nothing to disclose.
[a] Department of Otolaryngology, University of Minnesota, 516 Delaware Street Southeast, Suite 8-240, Minneapolis, MN 55455, USA; [b] Department of Otolaryngology, Paparella Ear Head & Neck Institute, University of Minnesota, 701, 25th Avenue South Suite 200, Minneapolis, MN 55454, USA
* Corresponding author.
E-mail address: dorri011@umn.edu

used a classification system to better describe the level of collapse seen in patients with OSA.[1] Type I describes abnormalities of the upper oropharyngeal airway, including the palate, uvula, and tonsils. Type II consist of upper oropharyngeal and hypopharyngeal airway pathology, and type III involves only the hypopharyngeal airway (lingual tonsils, tongue base, supraglottis, and hypopharynx). The importance of targeting the appropriate level of airway collapse is exemplified by Sher and colleagues,[2] who reported only a 5% success in patients with retrolingual (type II and III) collapse who undergo a uvulopalatopharyngoplasty (UPPP) alone. This article discusses a specific procedure designed to treat those patients with type II and type III obstruction.

Genioglossus advancement (GA) was first described by Riley and coworkers 1984.[3] The procedure involved the advancement of the genial tubercle/genioglossus muscle for the treatment of hypopharyngeal obstruction in OSA. The rationale of this technique was to stabilize the hypopharyngeal airway by moving forward the genioglossus complex providing tension on the base of the tongue and, thereby, expanding the airway in the anteroposterior dimension. Over the last 30 years, there have been variations proposed to the original technique to improve outcomes and limit complications.[4–7] Despite these variations, the principle of the procedure remains the same, and results have shown significant resolution of OSA symptoms and improvement in polysomnography data for those exhibiting type II (when combined with oropharyngeal procedures) and type III obstruction.

Understanding of GA begins at the anatomic level. The genioglossus muscle is an extrinsic muscle of the tongue. It originates from the superior mental spine or genial tubercles, and fans posterior to insert at the tip of the tongue, dorsum of the tongue, and into the body of the hyoid bone. This allows it to serve as a dilator of the pharynx at the level of the tongue base. The muscle is innervated by cranial nerve XII and receives its major vascular supply from the lingual arteries.

The anatomic dimensions of the musculature and its relationship to the anterior mandible are clinically significant to the GA. Studies have shown the width of the genial tubercle attachments to the inner table of the mandible can vary from 3 mm to 15 mm.[8,9] In the context of GA, understanding the proximity of the tubercle attachment to the tooth roots is also crucial. The superior border of the genial tubercle has been described, on average, just 6.45 mm inferior to the apex of the central incisor with 35% of specimens having less than 5 mm clearance from the incisor roots.[9] Understanding the anatomic relationship of the muscle to the anterior mandible and tooth roots helps the surgeon design an osteotomy for advancement of the tongue musculature. For maximal results, the dimensions of the osteotomy must be large enough to allow for the advancement of the greatest amount of genioglossus muscle without sacrificing the tooth roots.

The inferior border advancement genioplasty was the initial GA procedure described by Riley and colleagues.[3,4,7] The inferior border of the mandible is sectioned and advanced anteriorly with the dentoalveolar process left intact. The osteotomized segment must extend superiorly enough to incorporate the genioglossus attachment but not involve the tooth roots of the lower incisors or canines. Concerns regarding mandibular fracture led to minor innovations in the procedure by leaving an intact inferior mandible and advancing the genial tubercles anteriorly through a rectangular window osteotomy, as described by Li and colleagues (**Figs. 1** and **2**).[6,10]

Variations of this procedure include different types of osteotomies and slight alteration in transposition of the bone segment. The 90° rotation of the bony window segment involved in the previously stated procedure drew criticism for its risk of stripping the genial tubercle form the lingual cortex. An alternative technique involves a

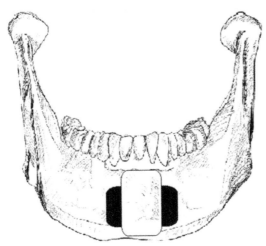

**Fig. 1.** Anterior view of the genioglossus advancement using the rectangular window technique.

similarly placed osteotomy with laterally slanting vertical cuts. The labial cortex and medullary bone are removed and the remaining lingual cortical bone (with intact genial tubercles) is then brought anteriorly without rotation and secured with a prebent plate.[5]

Garcia and colleagues[11] propose a slight alternative to the rectangular window by introducing a longitudinal groove on the floor of the window after the bony block is freed. The segment is then brought anterior and displaced inferiorly to overlap intact mandible in order for the genial tubercle to rest in the created groove. The advantages

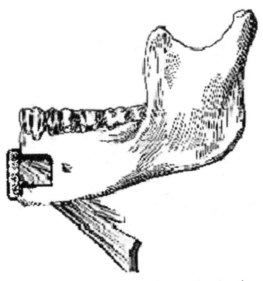

**Fig. 2.** Lateral view of the rectangular window technique showing the genioglossus attachments extending to the hyoid.

with this technique are greater anterior advancement of the genioglossus with inferior displacement and lack of segment rotation (avoiding possible stripping).[5,11] A circular trephination approach is also described, designed to reduce risk of lateral incisor tooth root injury while still maintaining optimal genial tubercle capture.[7,12]

In the patient with micrognathic OSA, further chin augmentation with mandibular advancement may be desired. In these instances a genioplasty combined with GA may be more appropriate. This is exemplified by Riley's original inferior border advancement genioplasty.[3] One may also consider a mortised genioplasty. The latter incorporates anterior advancement of the genioglossus, mylohyoid, digastric, and geniohyoid. This is accomplished in a similar method to the inferior mandibular osteotomy with the exception of the lateral cuts extending through the inferior border of the mandible and well lateral to the mental foramen.[8,13] Another option is a two-piece GA, described as a horizontal osteotomy mobilizing the inferior mandible segment in addition to the anterior rectangular window GA. This technique allows the direct visualization and palpation of the genioglossus after the inferior border of the mandible is reflected inferiorly. After the anterior rectangle block is advanced, the inferior border is reconstituted to improve the stability of the mandible and can be advanced antereriorly.[6] The GA can also be combined with hyoid elevation to increase the degree of hypopharyngeal airway expansion.[3,4,14–16] The hyoid is exposed and suspended with bilateral suture through the newly created bony window in the mandible.[16]

The combination of GA with other hypopharyngeal or oropharyngeal procedures is often necessary to fully address OSA, making direct comparisons between isolated procedures difficult. Although there is a paucity of level one and level two studies on the outcomes of GA for OSA, there have been numerous case series and retrospective studies with similarly positive results. Success, often described as apnea-hypopnea index (AHI) less than 20 and a 50% reduction of AHI, in the literature ranges widely between 40% and 70%.[14,15,17,18]

Riley and colleagues[17] described a 60% success rate out of 223 patients who received an UPPP and GA with hyoid suspension for type II upper airway obstruction. The study also showed 67% success in those who received only GA with hyoid suspension for type III obstruction, although there were only six patients in this group. "Success" in this study was defined as subjective and objective reports indicating significant improvement equivalent to that seen in patients monitored with nasal continuous positive airway pressure, or if the postoperative respiratory disturbance index (RDI) was less than 20 with at least a 50% reduction over the preoperative study. A review of the literature by Kezirian and Goldberg[19] revealed four case series totaling 91 cases and a success rate of 62%. Three of the four series showed a 67% to 78% success rate.

A prospective randomized study by Thomas and colleagues[20] comparing GA with tongue base suspension demonstrated a reduction in Epworth Sleepiness Scale (ESS) scores in the GA group (eight patients) from a mean of 13.3 to 5.4. Airway collapse for five of eight patients measured on Müller maneuver improved by a mean of 75% at the base of the tongue. Kuscu and colleagues[18] recently studied isolated GA results for patients and noted a 53% success rate; there was a significantly higher success rate for those with mild or moderate OSA compared with the severe cases, which is in line with other studies.[15]

Intraoperative complications of the various GA procedures include stripping of the genial tubercle from the lingual cortex of the bone segment, osseous segment necrosis, fracture of the labial cortex, fracture of the mandible, violation of tooth roots, and neurosensory changes.[5–7,11] The incidence of these complications seems to be low, but no systematic study has thoroughly evaluated this. The previous surgical technique discussion addresses the various alterations surgeons have proposed to decrease complication rates. Later complications include hematoma, seroma, infection, and mandible fracture; these too are rarely encountered.

There remains a critical role for hypopharyngeal procedures in the surgical treatment of OSA. GA is among the procedures designed for this subgroup of patients with OSA with collapse of the lower pharyngeal airway and shows consistently positive results. The surgical technique has evolved over the last 30 years and continues to be modified to increase its safety and efficacy. With careful patient selection, it remains a viable option in the surgical management of OSA.

## HYOID SUSPENSION PROCEDURES

Hyoid suspension is an adjuvant surgical therapy performed following or in combination with other surgical sleep procedures. The development of the procedure came about because patients had persistent upper airway obstruction and clinically evident sleep apnea after undergoing other procedures. Riley and colleagues[3,4] at Stanford University developed the initial surgical technique of hyoid suspension after noticing that patients who underwent UPPP did not have elimination of OSA. The group evaluated cephalometric roentgenograms of patients who failed UPPP and found that most of these patients had narrowing of pharyngeal airway at the base of the tongue.

Previous work in cephalometrics published by Riley and colleagues drew attention to three measurements: (1) pharyngeal airway space, (2) the length of the soft palate, and (3) the position of the hyoid bone. Patients with OSA demonstrated a trend toward having a more inferiorly displaced hyoid bone compared with control subjects. As would be expected, patients with mandibular deficiency were noted to have a significantly reduced pharyngeal airway space and none of them had elimination of OSA with UPPP.[21] Such patients have been shown to have improvement in OSA with total mandibular advancement. In mandibular advancement the pharyngeal airway is enlarged because of advancement of the genioglossus muscle and the base of tongue. Problems with mandibular advancement include the requirement of intermaxillary fixation and the change in dental occlusion.[4] The first procedure involving hyoid suspension that Riley and colleagues[4] developed addressed those patients that had a narrowed pharyngeal airway space by increasing the pharyngeal airway space without performing a formal mandibular advancement. The purpose of suspending the hyoid was to assist in stabilization of the mandibular osteotomy and to advance the tongue and subsequently further enlarge the pharyngeal airway.

The new technique was an inferior sagittal osteotomy of the mandible with hyoid myotomy and suspension. The mandible and hyoid are approached through a cervical incision. The mental nerves were identified and isolated and then an osteotomy was fashioned to include the genial tubercle to allow for advancement of the genioglossus muscle. The hyoid identified and the body and greater cornu are isolated and the sternohyoid, thyrohyoid, and omohyoid muscles are sectioned. Two strips of fascia lata were then placed around the body of the hyoid. The mandible fragment is moved anteriorly and stabilized with 24-gauge stainless steel wire. The hyoid is then moved anterosuperiorly and the fascia was fixed to the mandible with 26-gauge steel wire.[4] Correction of sleep apnea with this surgical procedure ranged from 60% to 70%.[3]

Additional work demonstrating the position of the hyoid and its effect on the pharyngeal airway was published by Van de Graaff and coworkers.[22] The group looked at the forces that act on the hyoid bone. They looked at airflow resistance in 12 dogs. The hyoid was displaced anteriorly either through manual anterior traction or through electrical stimulation. A significant reduction in airflow resistance was seen in both groups with inspiration and expiration. The conclusion was that in patients with OSA, obstruction at the level of the hypopharynx/base of tongue may be the result of decreased activity of the genioglossus and hyoid muscles.

Based on the results of Van DeGraff and coworkers,[22] which demonstrated a significant reduction in airway resistance with anterior displacement of the hyoid bone and that the cure rate of patients who underwent the inferior sagittal osteotomy of the mandible with hyoid myotomy and suspension was still only at 60% to 70%, Riley and colleagues[3] proposed a revised technique in hyoid suspension. The new technique involved dissection down to the level of the suprahyoid musculature followed by isolating a portion of the body of the hyoid at midline. An inferior myotomy is performed with the inferior border of the hyoid dissected clean while the suprahyoid musculature remains intact. The thyroid notch and the superior lamina are then identified. Ticron is then passed through the superior portion of the thyroid cartilage just lateral of midline bilaterally. It is placed around the hyoid bone and back through the thyroid cartilage. The resultant effect is anterior and inferior suspension of the hyoid bone over the thyroid cartilage.[3] In the first study that involved 15 patients who underwent the new technique, all underwent a UPPP and 14 underwent rectangular osteotomy and advancement of the genioglossus muscle. Each of the patients had persistent sleep apnea and therefore underwent the revised hyoid suspension procedure. Twelve of the patients had resolution of their excessive daytime sleepiness and had a significant polysomnographic improvement in their sleep-disordered breathing with a reduction of the RDI ($44.7 \pm 22.6$ to $12.8 \pm 6.9$). Of note, in one of the patients for whom the procedure was done under local anesthesia indirect laryngoscopy was performed and there was a significant improvement noted in the airway patency (**Fig. 3**).[3]

After Riley and colleagues developed the revised hyoid suspension, others have described various approaches to the technique. In 2004, Hörmann and Baisch[23]

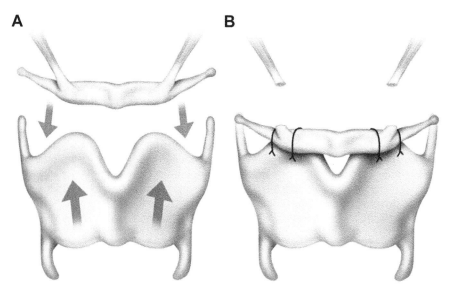

**A**  **B**

**Fig. 3.** (*A*) Release of hyoid attachments. (*B*) Inferior and anterior advancement of the hyoid over the thyroid cartilage. (*From* Pang KP, Terris DJ. Multilevel pharyngeal surgery for obstructive sleep apnea. In: Friedman M, editor. Sleep apnea and snoring. Philadelphia: Elsevier; 2009. p. 268–78; with permission.)

described their hyoid suspension technique. Dissection is taken down to the level of thyroid cartilage. Care is taken to disrupt as little of the perichondrium as to not disturb the blood supply to the thyroid cartilage. A sharp needle is then inserted through the thyroid cartilage. A steel 1-mm wire is then fixed at the end of the needle and the needle comes from posterior out of the contralateral side of the thyroid cartilage. The hyoid is then isolated and the steel wire is positioned around the hyoid. The hyoid is then moved inferiorly until it sits anterior to the thyroid cartilage. The two ends of the wire are then cinched to secure the hyoid in place (**Fig. 4**).

Medical device companies have also developed techniques for hyoid suspension. Medtronic (Minneapolis, MN) offers the AIRVance Hyoid Suspension system and Siesta Medical (Los Gatos, CA) offers the Encore Device for hyoid suspension. The two devices work in a similar fashion. As opposed to the revised hyoid suspension techniques previously described where the hyoid is suspended to the thyroid cartilage, both of these systems actually revert to the original process of hyoid suspension with suspension to the mandible. The surgical dissection then must include identification of the hyoid and the inner cortex of the mandible.

The Medtronic AIRVance Hyoid Suspension system uses a specially designed Airvance Bone Screw inserter to implant a screw into the posterior mandible approximately 1 to 1.5 cm up from the inferior rim at the level of the mandibular canines bilaterally. Sutures are fused to the bone screws. The hyoid is then advanced anteriorly and superiorly. The suture from bone screw on one side is then passed over a free needle and two passes around the hyoid from inferior to superior are made. The free needle is then passed to the suture on the contralateral side where two passes are made around the hyoid from superior to inferior. The sutures are then tied together in the midline effectively suspending the hyoid bone (**Fig. 5**).

In using the Siesta Medical Encore Device 1.5-mm holes are drilled bilaterally 1 cm to the midline in the inferoposterior mandible. Encore bone screws are then inserted into the predrilled holes. It is essential that the through hole on the bone screw is in an anteroposterior orientation. A specially designed lock tool is then used to loosen an internal lock screw and suture is removed. Suture is then placed in a specially

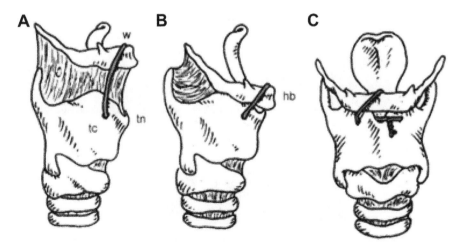

**Fig. 4.** The wire (*w*) is placed near the thyroid notch (*tn*) of the thyroid cartilage (*tc*) to avoid damage to the vocal cords. (*A*) Preoperative position of the hyoid bone (*hb*). (*B, C*) Position of the hyoid bone and the wire after surgical movement of the hyoid bone. (*From* Hormann K, Baisch A. The hyoid suspension. Laryngoscope 2004;114:1678; with permission.)

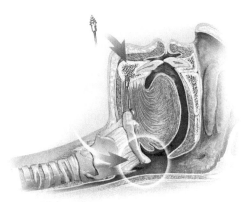

**Fig. 5.** Anterior and superior advancement of the hyoid with the use of the Medtronic AIRvance hyoid suspension system. (*Courtesy of* Medtronic, Minneapolis, MN; with permission.)

designed Revolution Suture Passer. This passer is then used to pass the suture from inferior to superior posterior to the hyoid bone. Two color-coded suture loops are then placed through the loop that was passed. These are all then pulled from superior to inferior behind the hyoid bone. Girth hitches are then placed around the mandible with the two color-coded sutures. A specially designed suture threader is then used to pass the suture through the corresponding bone screw. The hyoid is moved anterior and superior and the hyoid is suspended as the suture is locked into place in the bone screws (**Fig. 6**).

Hyoid suspension has been shown to be an effective adjuvant to other sleep surgical procedures in a multistep surgical approach to OSA.[19] The goal of hyoid

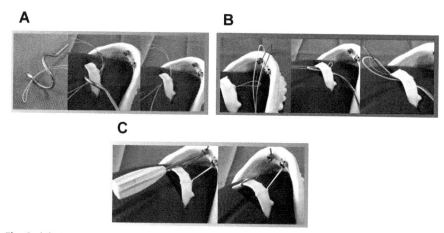

**Fig. 6.** (*A*) Siesta Medical Revolution Suture Passer is used to pass the suture from inferior to superior posterior to the hyoid bone. (*B*) Two color-coded suture loops are then placed through the loop that was passed by the Revolution Suture Passer. (*C*) The suture is locked into place in the bone corresponding bone screws. (*Courtesy of* Siesta Medical, Los Gatos, CA; with permission.)

suspension is anterior displacement of the hyoid resulting in increased patency of the hypopharyngeal airway and reduction of airway resistance. It has been shown to improve the likelihood of success in polysomnographic improvement in OSA when done in combination with other surgical sleep procedures. There are many acceptable methods for achieving adequate hyoid suspension (**Fig. 7**).

## TONGUE BASE PROCEDURES FOR OBSTRUCTIVE SLEEP APNEA

Since Fujita's original description of three airway types, many surgeons have realized that a significant majority of patients with OSA exhibit multilevel obstruction of the airway, with primary site being at the level of the tongue base. Many of these patients were found to have true macroglossia, whereas others had primarily prominent lingual tonsils or prominent musculature at the base of tongue. Moore and Phillips[24] further classified base of tongue obstruction as high tongue base type A, high tongue base with retroepiglottic narrowing type B1, type B2 diffuse tongue base narrowing, and type C isolated retroepiglottic narrowing. However, most of the newer surgical OSA procedures have been concentrating on the palatal obstruction. We have been able to define physiologic aspects of obstruction at the level of hard and soft palate, understand muscle dynamics of the area, and apply this knowledge to our surgical approaches. Surgical approaches to the tongue, even though performed for many years and well supported by the literature, still remain controversial. Therefore, tongue procedures for OSA have used various tools including traditional diathermy, lasers, radiofrequency (RF) probes, and coblation plasma technology, administered by human hand and robotically assisted. Extent of volumetric tongue reduction also varies from simple RF channeling to lingual tonsillectomy, midline partial glossectomy with or without associated linguoplasty, or even more extended posterior glossectomy.

First trials of conservative RF channeling at 460 kHz for sleep-disordered breathing were performed on porcine tongue by the group out of Stanford. Powell and colleagues[25] showed safe and successful tongue volume reduction by up to 26.3%. Based on that feasibility study of RF technology, the same group also did the first human trials with a remarkable success of reducing AHI by 55% and improving $O_2$ nadir by 12%.[26] Each study patient had multiple RF treatments (mean, 5.5) at 4-week intervals with total energy delivered into treatment zone of 8490 J. MRI demonstrated

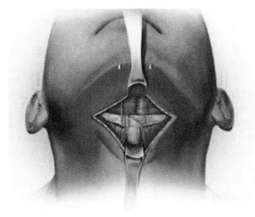

**Fig. 7.** Hyoid suspension.

tongue volume reduction of 17% and posterior pharyngeal space enlargement by 15% with minimal complications (1 tongue abscess out of 181 treatments). Thus, a new procedure was born (tongue base RF ablation) to manage retroglossal obstruction. This procedure could be implemented in an outpatient setting.

When the same authors from the Stanford group revisited their original pilot study 3 years later to evaluate long-term outcomes of RF tongue base reduction, the data from 16 out of original 18 patients were reexamined.[27] Even though there seemed to be long-term deterioration of AHI and RDI as compared with initial posttreatment values, there was still sustained improvement in both measures and continued decline in apnea index. There was a notable persistence in the improvement of patient quality of life measures (Short Form-36) and subjective sleepiness (as measured by the ESS).

Steward and colleagues[28] further demonstrated direct relationship between the number of temperature-controlled RF treatments and improved outcomes in patients with OSA. Increasing treatments from three to five per patient provided further improvement in OSA-related quality of life, snoring (SNORE 25), sleepiness, and median reaction time measurements in patients with mild to moderate sleep apnea.

Fibbi and colleagues[29] compared tongue base suspension with RF volumetric reduction, and found both techniques to be equally effective in significantly reducing the AHI ($P<.05$). Subjective sleepiness, assessed via ESS, also improved in both groups. However, just like in many other studies, there was a significant decrease in efficacy for both procedures as assessed by the previously mentioned parameters within 2 years of initial intervention.

Conclusions from a literature review meta-analysis of RF ablation of the tongue base for OSA in 2008 by Farrar and colleagues[30] support this procedure as a clinically effective tool in reducing ESS scores and RDI. Complications of the procedure, such as hematoma, abscess, and mucosal ulceration, were quite infrequent in most studies. Technologies that seem to be most commonly used to create thermal lesions in the tongue are bipolar RF and coblation (**Fig. 8**).

The procedure begins with a Peridex (3M, St Paul, MN) oral rinse, followed by a topical anesthetic, and then a local anesthetic infiltration. Using 22-gague RF needle electrode with a protective sheath (different products are available for the surgeon, although Gyrus ENT (Somnus Medical Technologies, Bartlett, TN) wands were extensively used in most of the studies), the tip is introduced submucosally not to exceed the depth of 20 mm to avoid potential damage to the hypoglossal neurovascular bundle located about 2 to 2.5 cm deep to the tongue dorsum. Extra vigilance has to be exercised to avoid superficial mucosal ulcerations delivering RF deep into genioglossus. Sites of therapy usually include midline and paramedian base of tongue, around and posterior to circumvallate papillae. Typical treatment zone ranges from 2.5 to 3 cm in diameter. With each entry of the electrode 600 to 750 J is delivered at 85° centigrade (**Fig. 9**).

The initial description of glossectomy by Fujita and coworkers[31] on 12 patients using the $CO_2$ laser reduced the RDI by more than 50% in 42% of patients. The RDI in responders decreased from 50.2 to 8.6. Two different studies combining UPPP and midline glossectomy demonstrated a success rate of 60%, defined as a reduction in RDI or AHI of more than 50%.[32,33] In a study combining midline laser glossectomy and extended uvuopalatal flap, an 83.3% success rate was reported, defined as a decrease in RDI to less than 20 and greater than 50% decrease.[34] A study combining midline glossectomy and epiglottidectomy in morbidly obese patients who had failed palatal surgery showed an overall success rate of 25%, defined as a decrease in RDI to less than 20. However the RDI of responders decreased from 69.7 to 10.[35] Woodson and Fujita,[36] using a technique described as a lingualplasty in a group of patients

A

B

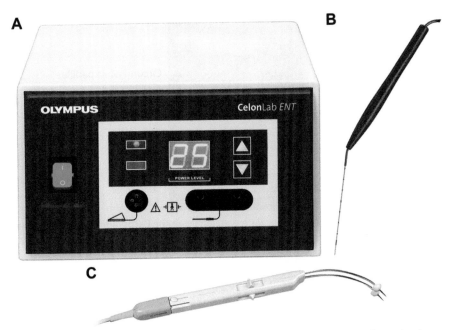

C

**Fig. 8.** (*A, B*) Bipolar radiofrequency Olympus Celon device with tongue base tip shown. (*C*) Gyrus radiofrequency bipolar tip. (*Courtesy of* Olympus, Center Valley, PA; with permission.)

who previously failed UPPP, demonstrated a 67% success rate, defined as a decrease in RDI to less than 20. Hou and colleagues[37] performed midline glossectomy and UPPP in 34 patients resulting in an improvement in AHI outcome by 74%, assessed 5 years postoperatively.

Techniques of controlled tongue base removal using a plasma wand device under endoscopic visualization, to obtain significant volumetric tongue base reduction, have been described. These include a submucosal minimally invasive lingual excision procedure introduced by Maturo and Mair initially for the treatment of pediatric macroglossia and later extrapolated to adults and open approaches.[38–40] In a study of 48 patients using the submucosal minimally invasive lingual excision approach, 65% of patients had successful AHI outcome.[41] The open approach of plasma wand glossectomy combined with palatoplasty in 39 patients resulted in AHI decrease from 49 to 19 and in another study performed on 50 patients the AHI declined from 52 to 18.[42,43] In a study of 27 patients who underwent midline glossectomy with lingualplasty using plasma wand or laser, and concurrent palatopharyngoplasty, the AHI was reduced from 44 to 13, with a reported success of 74%.[44] As surgeons became more comfortable with extensive resection of the anterior and posterior base of tongue, knowledge of the crucial anatomic relationships in the area gained even greater importance. In 1997 Lauretano and colleagues[45] demonstrated the relationship of the hypoglossal/lingual artery neurovascular bundle to the soft tissue and bony landmarks around the base of the tongue. They found that the neurovascular bundle was located 2.7 cm inferior and 1.66 cm lateral to the foramen cecum, 0.9 cm superior to the hyoid, 2.77 cm inferior and 1.1 cm medial to the lateral

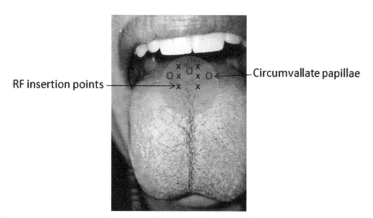

**Fig. 9.** Treatment area around circumvillate papillae using the Gyrus radiofrequency bipolar tip (**Fig. 8C**).

tongue margin at the level of foramen cecum, and 2.18 cm medial to the mandible at the level of retromolar trigone.

In this era of extensively used coblation-based bipolar plasma devices (Smith & Nephew ENT, Andover, MA), conservative lingual tonsillectomy may be extended to midline partial glossectomy performed with the Evac or Procise wands (**Fig.10**). Using 30° nasal endoscope or even a 5-mm 30° laparoscope with a nasotracheal tube in place offers excellent visualization of upper tongue base. Restricting tissue removal to the region medial to the neurovascular bundle reduces the rate of significant complications. The surgeon may wish to relinquish greater precision of dissection with needle tip diathermy for significantly less heat transfer to the surrounding tissues using coblation. Midline partial glossectomy may be performed in conjunction with linguoplasty if the aim is also to address macroglossia in the lateral extent of the tongue.

Recently a group from Australia described an operation that involved a classic midline glossectomy with linguoplasty combined with coblation-assisted channeling of the lateral tongue.[46] Four entries were created on each side of the junction of the dorsal and lateral tongue in the axial plane aiming the wand toward the circumvallate papillae. An important change in the technique of glossectomy was the addition of Harmonic focus curved shears (Ethicon Endo-surgery, Somerville, NJ) to resect the midline tongue segment to reduce heat transfer of traditional diathermy. No significant postoperative morbidity was noted in four patients treated with this technique.

A new study by Kim and colleagues[47] looking at obese adults may shed some light on predilection to sleep-disordered breathing based on fat deposition in the tongue. MRI findings in obese individuals with OSA demonstrated significantly greater tongue volumes as compared with obese control subjects caused by increased fat deposition especially toward the base of the tongue in the retroglossal space. Perhaps strategic fat ablation in the tongue using proper tools will prove beneficial to the volumetric expansion of the hypopharyngeal airway. This discovery merits further studies in this area.

As the human tongue is recognized for its role in oropharyngeal and hypopharyngeal obstruction in patients with OSA, various techniques of volumetric reduction of this structure have been attempted. All of these approaches have been supported by

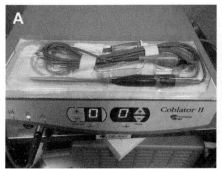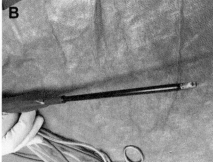

**Fig. 10.** Coblator. (*A*) Coblator system. (*B*) Coblator hand piece. (Images courtesy of Smith & Nephew, Inc.)

the literature for their positive impact in the reduction of AHI and minimal operative morbidity and long-term complications.

## REFERENCES

1. Fairbanks DNF. Snoring and obstructive sleep apnea. New York: Raven Press; 1987.
2. Sher AE, Schechtman KB, Piccirillo JF. The efficacy of surgical modifications of the upper airway in adults with obstructive sleep apnea syndrome. Sleep 1996; 19(2):156–77.
3. Riley R, Guilleminault C, Powell N, et al. Mandibular osteotomy and hyoid bone advancement for obstructive sleep apnea: a case report. Sleep 1984;7(1): 79–82.
4. Riley RW, Powell NB, Guilleminault C. Inferior sagittal osteotomy of the mandible with hyoid myotomy-suspension: a new procedure for obstructive sleep apnea. Otolaryngol Head Neck Surg 1986;94(5):589–93.
5. Demian NM, Alford J, Takashima M. An alternative technique for genioglossus muscle advancement in phase I surgery in the treatment of obstructive sleep apnea. J Oral Maxillofac Surg 2009;67(10):2315–8.
6. Li KK, Riley RW, Powell NB, et al. Obstructive sleep apnea surgery: genioglossus advancement revisited. J Oral Maxillofac Surg 2001;59(10):1181–4 [discussion: 1185].
7. Lee NR, Madani M. Genioglossus muscle advancement techniques for obstructive sleep apnea. Atlas Oral Maxillofac Surg Clin North Am 2007; 15(2):179–92.
8. Silverstein K, Costello BJ, Giannakpoulos H, et al. Genioglossus muscle attachments: an anatomic analysis and the implications for genioglossus advancement. Oral Surg Oral Med Oral Pathol Oral Radiol Endod 2000;90(6):686–8.
9. Mintz SM, Ettinger AC, Geist JR, et al. Anatomic relationship of the genial tubercles to the dentition as determined by cross-sectional tomography. J Oral Maxillofac Surg 1995;53(11):1324–6.
10. Li KK. Surgical therapy for obstructive sleep apnea syndrome. Semin Respir Crit Care Med 2005;26(1):80–8.

11. Garcia Vega JR, de la Plata MM, Galindo N, et al. Genioglossus muscle advancement: a modification of the conventional technique. J Craniomaxillofac Surg 2014; 42(3):239–44.

12. Miller FR, Watson D, Boseley M. The role of the genial bone advancement trephine system in conjunction with uvulopalatopharyngoplasty in the multilevel management of obstructive sleep apnea. Otolaryngol Head Neck Surg 2004; 130(1):73–9.

13. Hendler BH, Costello BJ, Silverstein K, et al. A protocol for uvulopalatopharyngoplasty, mortised genioplasty, and maxillomandibular advancement in patients with obstructive sleep apnea: an analysis of 40 cases. J Oral Maxillofac Surg 2001;59(8):892–7 [discussion: 898–9].

14. Ramirez SG, Loube DI. Inferior sagittal osteotomy with hyoid bone suspension for obese patients with sleep apnea. Arch Otolaryngol Head Neck Surg 1996;122(9): 953–7.

15. Vilaseca I, Morello A, Montserrat JM, et al. Usefulness of uvulopalatopharyngoplasty with genioglossus and hyoid advancement in the treatment of obstructive sleep apnea. Arch Otolaryngol Head Neck Surg 2002;128(4):435–40.

16. Wirtz N, Hamlar D. Genioglossus advancement for obstructive sleep apnea. Operative Techniques in Otolaryngology 2015;26(4):193–6.

17. Riley RW, Powell NB, Guilleminault C. Obstructive sleep apnea syndrome: a surgical protocol for dynamic upper airway reconstruction. J Oral Maxillofac Surg 1993;51(7):742–7 [discussion: 748–9].

18. Kuscu O, Suslu AE, Ozer S, et al. Sole effect of genioglossus advancement on apnea hypopnea index of patients with obstructive sleep apnea. Acta Otolaryngol 2015;135(8):835–9.

19. Kezirian EJ, Goldberg AN. Hypopharyngeal surgery in obstructive sleep apnea: an evidence-based medicine review. Arch Otolaryngol Head Neck Surg 2006; 132(2):206–13.

20. Thomas AJ, Chavoya M, Terris DJ. Preliminary findings from a prospective, randomized trial of two tongue-base surgeries for sleep-disordered breathing. Otolaryngol Head Neck Surg 2003;129(5):539–46.

21. Riley RW, Guilleminault C, Herran J, et al. Cephalometric analyses and flow loops in obstructive sleep apnea patients. Sleep 1983;6:303–11.

22. Van de Graaff WB, Gottfried SB, Mitra J, et al. Respiratory function of hyoid muscles and hyoid arch. J Appl Physiol Respir Environ Exerc Physiol 1984;57(1): 197–204.

23. Hormann K, Baisch A. The hyoid suspension. Laryngoscope 2004;114:1677–9.

24. Moore KE, Phillips C. A practical method for describing patterns of tongue-base narrowing (modification of Fujita) in awake adult patients with obstructive sleep apnea. J Oral Maxillofac Surg 2002;60(3):252–60.

25. Powell NB, Riley RW, Troell RJ, et al. Radiofrequency volumetric reduction of the tongue base: a porcine pilot study for the treatment of obstructive sleep apnea syndrome. Chest 1997;111:1348–55.

26. Powell NB, Riley RW, Guilleminault C. Radiofrequency tongue base reduction in sleep disordered breathing: a pilot study. Otolaryngol Head Neck Surg 1999; 120(5):656–64.

27. Li KK, Powell NB, Riley RW, et al. Temperature-controlled radiofrequency tongue base reduction for sleep-disordered breathing: long term outcomes. Otolaryngol Head Neck Surg 2002;127(3):230–4.

28. Steward DL, Weaver EM, Woodson BT. A comparison of radiofrequency treatment schemes for obstructive sleep apnea syndrome. Otolaryngol Head Neck Surg 2004;130(5):579–85.
29. Fibbi A, Ameli F, Brachetti F, et al. Tongue base suspension and radiofrequency volume reduction: a comparison between two techniques for the treatment of sleep-disordered breathing. Am J Otolaryngol 2009;30(6): 401–6.
30. Farrar J, Ryan J, Oliver E, et al. Radiofrequency ablation for the treatment of obstructive sleep apnea: a meta-analysis. Laryngoscope 2008;118(10):1878–83.
31. Fujita S, Woodson BT, Clark JL, et al. Laser midline glossectomy as a treatment for obstructive sleep apnea. Laryngoscope 1991;101(8):805–9.
32. Elasfour A, Miyazaki S, Itasaka Y, et al. Evaluation of uvulopalatopharyngoplasty in treatment of obstructive sleep apnea syndrome. Acta Otolaryngol Suppl 1998; 537:52–6.
33. Andsberg U, Jessen M. Eight years of follow-up-uvuloplatopharyngoplasty combined with midline glossectomy as a treatment for obstructive sleep apnea syndrome. Acta Otolaryngol Suppl 2000;543:175–8.
34. Li HY, Wang PC, Hsu CY, et al. Same-stage palatopharyngeal and hypopharyngeal surgery for severe obstructive sleep apnea. Acta Otolaryngol 2004;124(7): 820–6.
35. Mickelson SA, Rosenthal L. Midline glossectomy and epiglottidectomy for obstructive sleep apnea syndrome. Laryngoscope 1997;107(5):614–9.
36. Woodson BT, Fujita S. Clinical experience with lingualplasty as part of the treatment of severe obstructive sleep apnea. Otolaryngol Head Neck Surg 1992; 107(1):40–8.
37. Hou J, Yan J, Wang B, et al. Treatment of obstructive sleep apnea-hypopnea syndrome with combined uvulopalatopharyngoplasty and midline glossectomy: outcomes from a 5-year study. Respir Care 2012;57(12):2104–10.
38. Maturo SC, Mair EA. Submucosal minimally invasive lingual excision: an effective, novel surgery for pediatric tongue base reduction. Ann Otol Rhinol Laryngol 2006;115(8):624–30.
39. Robinson S, Lewis R, Norton A, et al. Ultrasound-guided radiofrequency submucosal tongue-base excision for sleep apnoea: a preliminary report. Clin Otolaryngol 2003;28:341–5.
40. Woodson BT. Innovative technique for lingual tonsillectomy and midline posterior of glossectomy for obstructive sleep apnea. Otolaryngol Head Neck Surg 2007; 18(1):20–8.
41. Friedman M, Soans R, Gurpinar B, et al. Evaluation of submucosal minimally invasive lingual excision technique for treatment of obstructive sleep apnea/hypopnea syndrome. Otolaryngol Head Neck Surg 2008;139(3):378–84.
42. Woodson BT, Laohasiriwong S. Lingual tonsillectomy and midline posterior glossectomy of obstructive sleep apnea. Otolaryngol Head Neck Surg 2012;23(2): 155–61.
43. Suh GD. Evaluation of open midline glossectomy in the multilevel surgical management of obstructive sleep apnea syndrome. Otolaryngol Head Neck Surg 2013;148(1):166–71.
44. Gunawardena I, Robinson S, MacKay S, et al. Submucosal lingualplasty for adult obstructive sleep apnea. Otolaryngol Head Neck Surg 2013;148(1):157–65.
45. Lauretano AM, Li KK, Caradonna DS, et al. Anatomic location of the tongue base neurovascular bundle. Laryngoscope 1997;107(8):1057–9.

46. MacKay SG, Jefferson N, Grundy L, et al. Coblation-assisted Lewis and MacKay operation(CobLAMO): new technique for tongue reduction in sleep apnoea surgery. J Laryngol Otol 2013;127(12):1222–5.
47. Kim AM, Keenan BT, Jackson N, et al. Tongue fat and its relationship to obstructive sleep apnea. Sleep 2014;37(10):1639–48.

# Transoral Robotic Partial Glossectomy and Supraglottoplasty for Obstructive Sleep Apnea

CrossMark

Mark A. D'Agostino, MD[a,b,c,d,e,*]

## KEYWORDS

- Sleep apnea • Obstructive sleep apnea • Treatment • Surgery • Robotic • TORS
- Base of tongue

## KEY POINTS

- The standard treatment for patients with obstructive sleep apnea syndrome is positive airway pressure (PAP) therapy (continuous PAP, bilevel PAP, auto titrating CPAP).
- Alternative therapies for patients who cannot tolerate PAP therapy include the use of oral appliances or upper airway surgery. The base of tongue plays an important role in this obstruction, and addressing the tongue base surgically can be a challenge for the head and neck surgeon.
- Transoral robotic surgery (TORS) using the da Vinci Surgical System provides a safe and effective way to approach and manage the base of tongue and supraglottis.
- TORS surgery offers clear advantages over alternative endoscopic and open procedures. These advantages include wide-field high-definition 3-D visualization, precise instrumentation, and when compared with open procedures, less operative time, quicker recovery, no external scars and comparable tissue resection.

## INTRODUCTION

Patients with obstructive sleep apnea (OSA) who fail positive airway pressure (PAP) therapy (continuous PAP [CPAP], bilevel PAP [BiPAP], auto titrating CPAP [AutoPAP]) may be considered for oral appliance therapy or surgery. Surgery may be used to augment CPAP compliance (by lowering pressure requirements) or in some cases

[a] Southern New England Ear, Nose and Throat Group, One Long Wharf Drive Suite 302, New Haven, CT 06511, USA; [b] Section of Otolaryngology, Department of Surgery, Yale University School of Medicine, 333 Cedar Street, New Haven, CT 06510, USA; [c] Department of Surgery, Frank H Netter School of Medicine, Quinnipiac University, 370 Bassett Road, North Haven, CT 06473, USA; [d] Department of Surgery, F. Edward Hebert School of Medicine, Uniformed Services University of the Health Sciences, 4301 Jones Bridge Road, Bethesda, MD 20814, USA; [e] Section of Otolaryngology, Department of Surgery, Middlesex Hospital, 28 Crescent Street, Middletown, CT 06457, USA
* One Long Wharf Drive, Suite 302, New Haven, CT 06511.
E-mail address: madago@comcast.net

Otolaryngol Clin N Am 49 (2016) 1415–1423
http://dx.doi.org/10.1016/j.otc.2016.07.009
oto.theclinics.com

may offer complete resolution of the apnea. Historically, many patients undergoing palatal procedures alone have been found to have residual apnea and considered surgical failures. The base of tongue has been proven to play a significant role in upper airway obstruction in many patients, and a main reason for failure of palatal procedures performed in isolation. Supplementing palatal procedures with procedures that address the hypopharynx and specifically the base of tongue can significantly improve surgical success rates in patients with OSA.[1] Standard procedures to address the tongue base include mandibular advancement, genioglossal advancement, hyoid suspension, tongue suspension, or base of tongue resection performed endoscopically as in a partial midline glossectomy or a tongue base reduction with hyoid epiglottoplasty, an open procedure described by Chabolle and colleagues.[2]

Weinstein and colleagues[3] and O'Malley and colleagues[4] pioneered transoral robotic surgery (TORS) using the da Vinci robotic system (Intuitive Surgical, Sunnyvale, CA) for minimally invasive transoral resection of oropharyngeal cancers, and in 2009 the Food and Drug Administration (FDA) approved TORS for benign and malignant lesions of the tongue base. This technique was extended to transoral resection of the base of tongue and supraglottoplasty in patients with OSA by Vincini and others,[5] and in 2014 the FDA approved TORS procedures for benign base of tongue resection procedures, after its safety and feasibility in patients with OSA were demonstrated.[6]

## PREOPERATIVE SELECTION

Potential surgical candidates should have OSA diagnosed by polysomnography and have failed positive pressure therapy (CPAP, BiPAP, or AutoPAP), the standard treatment for OSA. Patients also should have retrolingual collapse from a prominent base of tongue and/or prominent lingual tonsillar tissue as evident on fiberoptic endoscopic examination with Mueller maneuver in the office, or with drug-induced sleep endoscopy (DISE). DISE also can help identify patients whose obstruction is secondary to epiglottic collapse. Patients who have not tried CPAP or are compliant and well controlled with CPAP should not be considered for surgical intervention. Other contraindications to TORS base of tongue surgery would include patients with small oral cavities, trismus, or limited ability to open the mouth (interincisive distance <2.5 cm). Consideration also must be taken in patients with cervical problems and limited ability to extend the head and neck. Patients with any degree of dysphagia (unless the dysphagia is secondary to lingual tonsillar hypertrophy), swallowing complaints, psychiatric illnesses, or have an ASA greater than 3 should also not be considered for a robotic partial glossectomy.

## ANATOMIC CONSIDERATIONS

One must be familiar with the anatomy of the tongue base, which when viewed transorally, is quite different from the usual lateral approach most head and neck surgeons are used to. The neurovascular structures are lateral and deep within the tongue musculature; therefore, dissection in the midline involving the intrinsic tongue muscles is safe. The main trunk of the lingual artery, a branch of the external carotid artery, lies on the lateral surface of the genioglossus muscle and is covered by the hyoglossus muscle. The artery runs along the greater cornu of the hyoid bone, and then passes below the hyoglossus muscle where it gives off the dorsal lingual arteries for the tongue base and the deep lingual branches to the body of the tongue. The hypoglossal nerve and vein are more lateral and lie on the external surface of the hyoglossus muscle. The glossopharyngeal nerve runs along the lateral surface of the stylopharyngeus muscle, and at the level of the tongue base splits into branches for the tongue base and tonsillar region, making identification of this nerve much more difficult when viewed transorally.[7]

## OPERATIVE TECHNIQUE

All procedures are performed under general anesthesia. Patients undergo either orotracheal or nasotracheal intubation. Intravenous steroids and a broad spectrum antibiotic are given. The patient is placed in a "sniffing" positon, and the bed is rotated away from the anesthesiologist 90° to 180°. Protective eye goggles and mandibular and maxillary dentition guards are placed. A 0–silk suture is placed in the midline of the tongue to aid in retraction out of the oral cavity (**Fig. 1**). There are several oral retractors that may be used. A commonly used oral retractor is the FK retractor (Gyrus, Gyrus Medical, Maple Grove, Minnesota) (**Figs. 2** and **3**), although the author's preference is a Crowe Davis mouth gag (Karl Storz, Tuttlingen, Germany) with Davis Meyer blades (**Fig. 4**). The Davis Myer blades are flat (no indentation for the endotracheal tube) and have a suction port at the distal tip. The blades come in half sizes, which is helpful. Best exposure is often obtained with a short but wide tongue blade. A retractor holder that attaches to the bed frame is most helpful. The da Vinci robot is docked along the right side of the bed and the arms are loaded with two 5-mm Endowrists, a Maryland Dissector used for grasping and retracting tissue, and a monopolar cautery with a spatula tip for dissection. The center arm is loaded with an 8.5-mm 30° high-definition 3-dimensional camera (a 12-mm camera may also be used). The camera provides a very clear and detailed high-definition 3-dimensional image, and offers the option of digital zoom. The robotic arms are extended over the patient's head and introduced into the oral cavity (**Fig. 5**). An assistant is seated at the head of the patient and helps with retraction, suctioning, and repositioning of the robotic arms in the event of collisions.

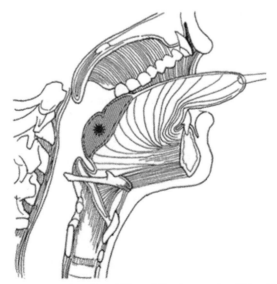

**Fig. 1.** A 0-silk suture is placed in the midline of the tongue to aid in retraction out of the oral cavity. The asterisk show the area of tongue base that should be resected. (*From* D'Agostino M. Transoral robotic partial glossectomy and supraglottoplasty for obstructive sleep apnea. Operat Tech Otolaryngol Head Neck Surg 2015;26(4):212; with permission.)

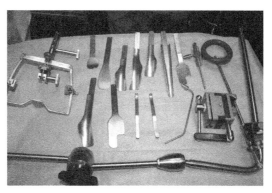

**Fig. 2.** Photo of FK retractor.

Standard fire precautions are taken, the $Fio_2$ should be kept below 30%, and suction Bovie and hemoclips are available on the back table should they be necessary. The surgeon is seated at the console. Landmarks should be identified: the circumvallate papillae, foramen cecum, vallecula, and epiglottis. In some patients, it may be difficult to visualize the epiglottis at the start of the procedure, but it should certainly be seen as the dissection progresses. The procedure is begun by removing the lymphatic tissue from the base of the tongue first on the right side and then on the left. Dissection is carried out just posterior from the circumvallate papillae, down into the vallecula and across to the base of the epiglottis dissecting the lymphatic tissue off of the underlying musculature (**Fig. 6**). It is often easier to perform a midline split of the lymphatic tissue from the foramen cecum down to the base of the epiglottis (**Fig. 7**), and remove the right and left sides separately. The procedure is then repeated on the left side. Hemostasis is obtained during the dissection and great care is taken laterally to avoid the lingual artery and its branches. Once the lymphatic tissue has been removed (**Fig. 8**), the procedure is repeated, removing a layer of muscle across the tongue base (up to 10 mm), right and then left side, and if necessary, an additional strip of muscle (up to 5 mm) may be removed in the midline only, to avoid injury to the lingual nerve (**Fig. 9**). The tissue removed is quantified by measuring volume displacement in a syringe. The average amount of tissue removed is approximately 10 mL, depending on the individual, and studies have shown a trend toward the amount of tissue

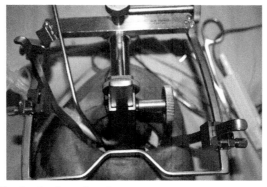

**Fig. 3.** Photo of FK retractor in oral cavity.

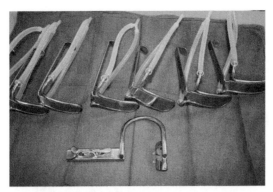

**Fig. 4.** Photo of Crowe Davis retractor.

removed and success.[8] Removal of less than 7 mL of tissue is likely insufficient for success, and greater than 20 mL of tissue removal is oftentimes not needed. Hemostatic agents are usually not necessary. In patients found to have epiglottic collapse on sleep endoscopy, an epiglottoplasty may be performed at this point. A vertical cut is made in the midline of the epiglottis down to, but not below, the level of the hyoid,

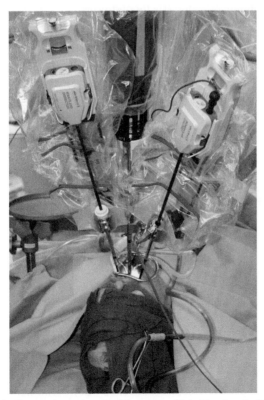

**Fig. 5.** Photo of robotic arms in oral cavity. (*Courtesy of* Intuitive Surgical Inc, Sunnyvale, CA; with permission.)

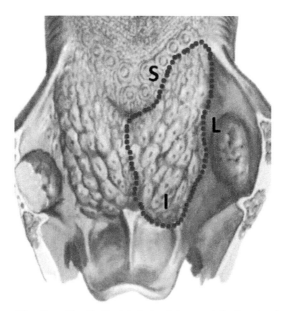

**Fig. 6.** Definition of the dissection limits. I, inferior (glossoepiglottic sulcus); L, lateral (amygdaloglossus sulcus); S, superior (sulcus terminalis). (*From* D'Agostino M. Transoral robotic partial glossectomy and supraglottoplasty for obstructive sleep apnea. Operat Tech Otolaryngol Head Neck Surg 2015;26(4):212; with permission.)

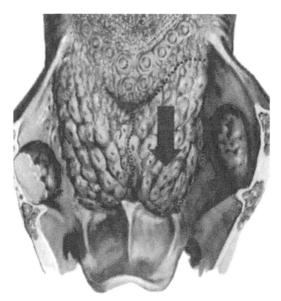

**Fig. 7.** Direction of lingual tonsil resection. (*From* D'Agostino M. Transoral robotic partial glossectomy and supraglottoplasty for obstructive sleep apnea. Operat Tech Otolaryngol Head Neck Surg 2015;26(4):212; with permission.)

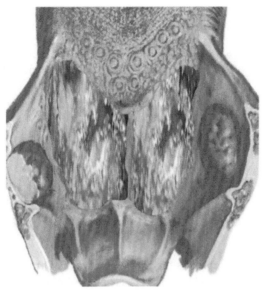

**Fig. 8.** Completed lingual tonsillectomy. (*From* D'Agostino M. Transoral robotic partial glossectomy and supraglottoplasty for obstructive sleep apnea. Operat Tech Otolaryngol Head Neck Surg 2015;26(4):212; with permission.)

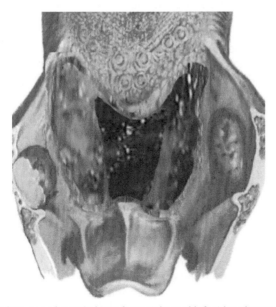

**Fig. 9.** Removal of 10 mm of muscle layer from right and left sides plus up to 5 mm of additional strip midline only. (*From* D'Agostino M. Transoral robotic partial glossectomy and supraglottoplasty for obstructive sleep apnea. Operat Tech Otolaryngol Head Neck Surg 2015;26(4):212; with permission. Figure 10.)

leaving at least a 5-mm stump. Horizontal cuts are then made on each side to the midline cut, thus removing a horizontal strip across the top of the epiglottis, leaving an epiglottic stump to prevent aspiration. Patients are usually extubated in the operating room and observed overnight in a monitored bed. If the airway is deemed to be too tenuous, the surgeon may prefer to leave the patient intubated, or perform a tracheostomy.

## POSTOPERATIVE CARE

Patients are observed overnight in a monitored bed and given intravenous steroids and antibiotics. They are started on a clear liquid diet that is advanced as tolerated. Most patients are discharged home on postoperative day 1 and sent home with oral antibiotics and a short steroid taper in addition to liquid analgesics. Pain, dysphagia, and dysgeusia usually resolve in 2 to 3 weeks, but may take longer in some patients.

## COMPLICATIONS

The most common complications include temporary dysphagia, dehydration hypogeusia, and limited late bleeding. Patients will often complain of difficulty swallowing and taste disturbance, both of which usually resolve by 2 to 3 weeks but can last longer or rarely be permanent. Late bleeding may be seen in 3% to 4% of cases (similar to tonsillectomy postoperative bleeding) and usually occurs 2 to 3 weeks postoperatively. This is often self-limited bleeding, but may require intervention in some cases. Occasionally patients may complain of temporary tongue numbness from paresis of the lingual nerve caused by pressure on the tongue from the mouth gag. This usually resolves in 2 to 4 weeks. Limiting the amount of time the mouth gag is in place and opened will help to avoid this problem. Other potential complications include tooth or lip injury, transient pharyngeal or supraglottic edema, or pharyngeal scarring. More severe complications include intraoperative bleeding from injury to the lingual artery or one of its branches, which may require opening the neck to gain control, loss of the airway, death, or paralysis of the hypoglossal nerve, which has not been reported. In a study by Hoff and colleagues[6] involving 293 TORS procedures for OSA, the complication rate was 20.7%. None of the complications were specifically related to the use of the da Vinci Surgical System, and none of the complications were life threatening: all complications were resolved by intervention and/or hospitalization. The most common complications were bleeding (4.1%), dehydration (4.8%), and dysphagia (5.1%) requiring intervention. In a series of 243 TORS procedures for OSA, Vincini and colleagues[9] reported transient and mild hypogeusia as the most common complication (14.2%) and a 5.0% bleed rate (2.9% late bleeding and self-limited, 1.7% requiring surgical intervention, and a 0.4% rate of significant intraoperative hemorrhage).

## RESULTS

A multicenter study reported by Vincini and colleagues[9] involving 243 patients undergoing multilevel surgery (14% underwent TORS only), a success rate of 66.9% was reported (success defined as a >50% reduction in apnea hypopnea index [AHI], with a final AHI <20, epworth sleepiness score [ESS] <10).

The author's experience of 50 patients undergoing multilevel surgery including TORS (of more than 100 TORS cases) demonstrated a success rate of 80% (defining success as a >50% reduction in AHI, and a final AHI <20).[7]

## SUMMARY

TORS using the da Vinci Surgical System offers an exceptional 3-dimensional view and exposure to the tongue base, with distinct advantages over other procedures used for tongue base resection, including both open and other transoral procedures. Although still in its infancy, early studies have demonstrated both safety and efficacy.

## REFERENCES

1. Kezirian EJ, Goldberg AN. Hypopharyngeal surgery in obstructive sleep apnea: an evidence-based medicine review. Arch Otolaryngol Head Neck Surg 2006; 132(2):206–13.
2. Chabolle F, Wagner I, Blumer MB, et al. Tongue base reduction with hyoepiglottoplasty: a treatment for severe obstructive sleep apnea. Laryngoscope 1999;109: 1273–80.
3. Weinstein GS, O'Malley BW Jr, Hockstein NG. Transoral robotic surgery: supraglottic laryngectomy in a canine model. Laryngoscope 2005;115:1315–9.
4. O'Malley BW Jr, Weinstein GS, Snyder W, et al. Transoral robotic surgery (TORS) for base of tongue neoplasms. Laryngoscope 2006;116:1465–72.
5. Vincini C, Dallan I, Canzi P, et al. Transoral robotic tongue base resection in obstructive sleep apnoea-hypopnoea syndrome: a preliminary report. ORL J Otorhinolaryngol Relat Spec 2010;72(1):22–7.
6. Hoff P, D'Agostino M, Thaler E. Transoral robotic surgery in benign diseases including obstructive sleep apnea: safety and feasibility. Laryngoscope 2015; 125(5):1249–53.
7. Dallan I, Seccia V, Faggioni L, et al. Anatomical landmarks for transoral robotic tongue base surgery: comparison between endoscopic, external and radiological perspectives. Surg Radiol Anat 2013;35:3–10.
8. D'Agostino M, Folk D, Adams S, et al. Transoral robotic surgery for obstructive sleep apnea. Presented at the Combined Otolaryngologic Society Spring Meetings. Las Vegas (NV). May 15, 2014.
9. Vincini C, Montevecchi F, Campanini A, et al. Clinical outcomes and complications associated with TORS for osahs: a benchmark for evaluating an emerging surgical technology in a targeted application for benign disease. ORL J Otorhinolaryngol Relat Spec 2014;76:63–9.

# Upper Airway Stimulation Therapy

Katherine Koral Green, MD, MS[a],*, B. Tucker Woodson, MD[b]

## KEYWORDS

- Obstructive sleep apnea • Sleep surgery • Hypoglossal nerve
- Cranial nerve stimulation

## KEY POINTS

- Obstructive sleep apnea (OSA) in adults is often a multifactorial process, with both mechanical and physiologic processes contributing to airway collapse during sleep.
- Contraction of the base of tongue provides support and stabilization of the posterior oropharynx through a complex interaction with the palate and oropharyngeal constrictors. This assists in maintaining a patent airway.
- Muscle tone during sleep is influenced by the loss of tonic muscle activity to the upper airway with sleep onset, $CO_2$-mediated ventilatory instability, and an inadequate activation of phasic genioglossus muscle reflex.
- Traditional surgical interventions for OSA address the mechanical (anatomic) contributions to OSA by altering soft tissue. The Inspire II implant is the first surgical intervention to address the physiologic processes that contribute to OSA.
- In a multicenter, prospective cohort study, patients were implanted with the Inspire II system and followed for 12 months. Apnea Hypopnea Index (AHI) decreased by 68% after implant, and 63% of patients had a postimplant AHI of less than 15 events per hour.

## INTRODUCTION

Upper airway stimulation acts to reduce or eliminate upper airway collapse and resultant obstructive sleep apnea (OSA) by augmenting genioglossus muscle tone during sleep. It is unique among surgical interventions in that it does not attempt to reconstruct the structure of the upper airway, but rather augments mechanisms of physiologic compensation to prevent OSA. A novel approach warrants an understanding of these processes.

[a] Department of Otolaryngology Head and Neck Surgery, University of Colorado School of Medicine, 12631 East, 17th Avenue MS B205, Aurora, CO 80045, USA; [b] Division of Sleep Medicine and Surgery, Department of Otolaryngology, Medical College of Wisconsin, 9200 W Wisconsin Ave, Milwaukee, WI 53226, USA
* Corresponding author.
*E-mail address:* katherine.green@ucdenver.edu

Otolaryngol Clin N Am 49 (2016) 1425–1431
http://dx.doi.org/10.1016/j.otc.2016.07.010
oto.theclinics.com

## MECHANISMS OF UPPER AIRWAY COLLAPSE AND PHYSIOLOGY OBSTRUCTIVE SLEEP APNEA

### Overview

Airway collapse in OSA is the result of a complex interaction of both upper airway structural characteristics and ventilatory physiology during sleep. It is an imbalance between a structurally smaller (and therefore at-risk) upper airway and physiologic mechanisms that sustain breathing during sleep. The contribution of these 2 processes is highly variable between individuals and results in vast differences in the underlying physiologic disturbance responsible for an individual's OSA. But the consequence of this imbalance is an upper airway that is unable to maintain adequate ventilation to sustain life.

### Anatomic Considerations

Multiple anatomic features contribute to the abnormal upper airway in OSA in adults. It is the common scenario that when combined they all contribute to a small upper airway, which when exposed to the stress of sleep onset and ventilatory (loop gain) instability leads to obstruction. Multiple structural phenotypes may exist that contribute to the risk of OSA.

### Tongue anatomy

The tongue is a vital muscle that is responsible for a variety of functions, from speech and mastication, to maintenance of a patent airway and pharyngeal stability. The anterior tongue is responsible for speech and mastication, while the posterior tongue is responsible for maintaining pharyngeal stability. In people, the posterior tongue anatomically is not in the oral cavity but is the anterior wall of the pharynx. The differences in these functions are highlighted by distinct differences in both the anatomy and physiology of the anterior and posterior tongue musculature.

The human tongue is comprised of 8 pairs of skeletal muscles: 4 paired extrinsic muscles (with a bony attachment to anchor the tongue and movements) and 4 paired intrinsic muscles, with no bony attachments. Extrinsic muscle fibers originate from external bony attachments and terminate in the tongue, whereas intrinsic muscles both originate and terminate within the tongue. As a general rule, whole-tongue movements are attributed to extrinsic muscle function, whereas lingual-shaped changes are attributed to intrinsic musculature. The posterior tongue muscles are significantly more fatigue resistant than those of the anterior fibers because of a higher percentage of slow-twitch type I fibers. This is similar to the fatigue-resistant composition of cardiac and diaphragmatic muscle fiber composition, which are designed to withstand fatigue and constant, sustained activity. The high ratio of fatigue-resistant fibers is critical for functions requiring sustained, tonic contractions, as is seen in swallowing and maintaining airway stability.

### Tongue-palate-oropharynx interaction

The anatomic and functional relationships between the tongue base and the superior pharyngeal constrictor and the tongue base and palate are key to understanding the potential benefit in using hypoglossal nerve stimulation to improve airway stability. The central third (the anterior wall) of the oropharynx is formed by the posterior aspect of the tongue. The superior pharyngeal constrictor muscle forms the muscular ring of the hypopharynx. Studies have shown that movements of the tongue create a forward mechanical drag on the superior constrictor muscle, which makes the pharyngeal wall stiffer and less compliant, therefore less prone to collapse. The stability of the oropharynx is not only dependent on the stiffness of the constrictor muscles themselves, but also in part depends on the stiffness of the posterior lingual muscles, although some of these are known tongue retractors. A similar, but less well understood relationship exists between the palate and the tongue. Velopharyngeal patency may be mediated by the palatoglossal arch, direct compressive effects of the tongue, or oropharyngeal surface interactions. Contractions of the tongue musculature, regardless of whether they are protrusive or retrusive functions, potentially stabilize and stiffen the palatoglossal fold by applying mechanical drag. In 2003, Isono and colleagues[1] examined the dynamic interaction between the posterior tongue and the soft palate in patients with sleep apnea. It was noted that a close apposition between the tongue and soft palate (the tongue–soft palate interface) occurred with variable magnitude in all patients with sleep-disordered breathing, and that there was a progressive increase in contact pressure between the tongue and soft palate during obstructive apneic events. This contributed to maintaining retropalatal closure. Release of this vector of force would assist in opening the palate in some patients. Finally, surface tension forces interact to contribute to upper airway collapse and reopening. Forward movements of the tongue may displace the palate, which is adherent by surface tension forces.

### Physiologic Considerations

No single physiologic process contributes to OSA. A major contributor to the transmural or stabilizing pressure of the upper airway is upper airway muscle tone. Muscle tone during sleep is influenced by: (1) the loss of tonic muscle activity to the upper airway with sleep onset, (2) loss of upper airway muscle tone due to $CO_2$-mediated ventilatory instability, and (3) an inadequate activation of phasic genioglossus muscle reflex. All are ultimately mediated by activity of the hypoglossal nerve (CN XII).

Historically, abnormal timing of the activation of the diaphragm and upper airway muscles was considered a major physiologic factor in OSA. The early onset of diaphragm contraction, which exposed the relatively passive upper airway to significant negative inspiratory forces, could potentially obstruct the airway. An earlier preactivation of the genioglossus muscle could preempt this and prevent obstruction.

Although asynchronous timing of upper and lower airway muscles does occur in sleep, it is more likely that the partial or complete loss of compensatory upper airway muscle tone is the major contributor to sleep apnea. This includes the sleep-related loss of the negative pressure-mediated genioglossus muscle reflex, the progressive loss of tonic muscle tone at sleep onset and with various sleep stages, and the massive changes in muscle tone (zenith and nadir) that occur due to the $CO_2$-mediated changes in ventilatory drive during nonrapid eye movement (non-REM) sleep. Upper airway stimulation (UAS) interacts with all these to reduce the propensity of the upper airway to obstruct.

## HISTORY OF UPPER AIRWAY STIMULATION

Conceptually, several hallmark studies were key in considering nerve stimulation as a treatment for OSA. Remmers and colleagues[2] suggested that pharyngeal obstruction resulted from disturbances in upper airway neuromuscular control during sleep. Since that time, it has been shown that at sleep onset, pharyngeal collapse is associated with loss of genioglossal tone,[3] but that reflexes exist that are activated by airway obstruction to increase pharyngeal tone and restore airway patency during sleep.[4,5] These ideas have served as the underlying theories with which people have pursued neural stimulation as a treatment for OSA.

Early animal models showed that exogenous stimulation of this muscle augmented the activity of this muscle and restored upper airway patency.[6] Histopathological evaluation revealed no significant nerve damage from chronic stimulation. Another animal study was used to evaluate the reversibility of inspiratory airflow limitations, comparing hypoglossal nerve stimulation to continuous positive airway pressure (CPAP). They found that hypoglossal nerve stimulation was as effective as CPAP in reversing both inspiratory flow limitation and snoring.[7]

Early pilot human studies looking at genioglossus stimulation trialed 3 different techniques: submental transcutaneous stimulation, direct fine wire stimulation, and direct hypoglossal nerve stimulation. Early studies with submental stimulation did document improvement in airflow and reductions in sleep apnea severity, but this technique resulted in frequent arousals and inconsistent results, thus making it an ineffective method of treatment. Similarly, transcutaneous stimulation resulted in stimulation of sensory nerves and inconsistent stimulation of motor neurons.[8]

Studies examining sublingual transmucosal and fine wire intramuscular electrodes noted that there was variability in response based on the location of the stimulus applied, with proximal stimulation activating the lingual retrusor muscles, and distal stimulation activating the genioglossus protrusor functions. Laboratory-based studies demonstrated that combined stimulation of these muscles, when paired with methods to improve ventilatory drive, served to stiffen the pharynx and not just move the tongue anteriorly. This combination maximally aided maintaining airway patency. However, although selective stimulation of multiple antagonistic muscle groups seemed to be of benefit, this has not been observed in clinical studies.

In 1997, Eisele and colleagues[9] published the first study on 5 implanted patients with hypoglossal nerve cuff electrodes. Stimulation was manually applied while asleep during partially obstructed inspirations and demonstrated significant increases in maximal inspiratory airflow. This study provided sufficient data to compel full development of an implantable hypoglossal nerve stimulating system.

### Inspire II Implant

The Inspire II implant (Inspire Medical, Maple Grove, MN) is an implantable UAS device that is targeted at increasing activity of the hypoglossal nerve during sleep. The device has multiple components, including an implantable pulse generator (IPG), sensing lead, stimulation lead, and physician and patient programmers. The IPG, sensing, and stimulation leads are all implanted at the time of surgery.

### Implantable Pulse Generator

The IPG includes the programming software, communication device, and battery for the system to function. The IPG is directly linked by electrode wires to the sensing and stimulation leads. Within the IPG software is the ability to program both triggers for the sensory lead and parameters for the stimulation lead. The IPG can communicate bidirectionally with the physician programmer, who may modulate all the programming modes. It unidirectionally communicates with the patient programmer and has on/off and limited programming for patient adjustments.

### Sensory Lead

The sensory lead is a differential pressure transducer that measures and senses changes in ventilatory pressures. It is surgically placed between the internal and external intercostal muscles to sense pleural pressure. To avoid cardiac artifact, it is placed on the right lateral chest.

## Stimulation Lead

The stimulation lead contains 3 electrodes in a flexible cuff that is placed around the hypoglossal nerve. The electrodes can be programmed in various unipolar and monopolar fashions. The device is implanted surgically under general anesthesia via 3 small incisions. The nerve stimulation lead is placed via a submandibular incision, which provides ready access to the hypoglossal nerve as it courses distal to the anterior belly of the diagastric muscle. The IPG is implanted into a subclavicular pouch superficial to the pectoralis muscle fascia. The sensing lead is placed via a midaxillary incision at the intercostal interspaces 4 or 5. A tunneling device allows for passage of electrode leads subcutaneously to the site of the IPG. Once implanted, the wounds are allowed to heal, and the device is activated 1 month after surgery.

## REVIEW OF PUBLISHED DATA

Clinical experience with an implantable human device was initiated in 1997 with the implantation of 8 patients in Europe and the United States using the Inspire TM 1 device. This device differed significantly from the currently approved device. The initial device included a sensing lead placed through a drill hole in the manubrium and into the mediastinum, placement of the stimulation lead on the main trunk of the hypoglossal nerve distal to the ansa cervicalis, and stimulation being applied at the onset of inspiration and limited to the inspiratory cycle. In addition, in the initial clinical experience, electrode wire fractures occurred in 5 of 8 patients requiring redesign of the stimulation electrode. Clinical results demonstrated that the device was well tolerated by patients and resulted in significant reduction in apnea severity. Non-REM AHI decreased from 52.0 to 20.4 events per hour, and REM AHI decreased from 48.2 to 30.5 events per hour. Subsequent physiologic and clinical studies performed on the patients provided physiologic information documenting improvements in airflow, lack of sleep fragmentation, and sensory stimulation that had been observed with methods that directly stimulated the upper airway muscles.

Several prospective, investigational studies have been performed examining the safety and efficacy of 2 devices, the Apnex Medical Hypoglossal Nerve Stimulation System and the Inspire II Upper Airway Stimulation System.

## Apnex

In 2011, an Australian prospective study was published on the Apnex HGNS system. This system is similar to the Inspire system in that it has a cuff electrode on the hypoglossal nerve, an IPG, and a sensing lead to coordinate with ventilation. This sensing lead uses chest wall impedance to determine phase of ventilation. Twenty-one patients were implanted and showed a significant improvement in AHI as well as several validated survey scores at 6 months compared with baseline. There was good compliance and consistent use of the device throughout the study.[10]

In 2012, Goding and colleagues[11] examined the anatomic changes seen with activation of the HGNS system, using fluoroscopy to examine the dimensions of the airway. All patients demonstrated anterior displacement of the tongue and an increase in the anterior–posterior retrolingual airway during stimulation.

Kezirian and colleagues[12] examined the safety, feasibility, and efficacy of the HGNS system. Thirty-one patients were implanted and had follow-up at 6 and 12 months. There were significant improvements in AHI severity and functional outcomes of sleep (FOSQ) when the 12-month follow-up values were compared with the cohort baseline. AHI severity went from 45.4 plus or minus 17.5 to 25.3 plus or minus 20.6 events per hour when comparing baseline to 12-month values. Apnex did not complete it's clinical trial for approval by the Food and Drug Administration (FDA), however, and is no longer commercially available. These early studies were key in identifying patient factors that were correlated with success of stimulation therapy.

### Inspire II

The Inspire II device is the first commercially available device UAS device approved by the FDA for the treatment of obstructive sleep apnea. In 2012, a pilot study was published examining the safety and preliminary effectiveness of Inspire II.[13] Part I of the study identified factors to predict best efficacy from implantation, and found that patients with a body mass index (BMI) less than 32 and an AHI less than 50 who did not have complete concentric palatal collapse were most likely to benefit from implantation. In the second part of the study, those criteria were used in patient selection, and 8 patients were implanted, with an improvement in AHI from 38.9 to 10.0 at 6 months after implantation.

More recently, a large, multicenter, prospective cohort study examined the efficacy and safety of the Inspire II UAS system.[14] One hundred twenty-two subjects with moderate or severe sleep apnea (AHI of >20 and < 50 events/h, BMI of <32 kg/m$_2$, and without concentric retropalatal collapse on drug induced sleep endoscopy) were implanted and followed for 1 year. The median AHI score decreased by 68% at 12 months after implant, from 29.3 to 9.0 events per hour. Sixty-six percent and 75% of the patients met the primary outcome definitions of success using AHI and oxygen desaturation index. Sixty-three percent had an AHI of less than 15 events per hour. Quality-of-life measures and sleepiness was normalized at 1 year in the group. Additionally, improvements in sleep stages and diastolic blood pressure were observed in the group at 12 months compared with baseline. The device-related serious complications occurred in 2 of 126 subjects and required repositioning of the implant. Device- and nondevice-related serious complications were less than 2%. Less serious complications included tongue discomfort or abrasions that were treated conservatively and substantially resolved and did not require device use cessation.

In 46 successfully treated patients, a randomized therapy withdrawal trial was performed after 12 months.[15] In this group, the withdrawal group returned to pretreatment disease levels, while the group with therapy maintained did not change and remained successful. Prospective outcomes continue to be collected for this initial Stimulation Therapy for Apnea Reduction (STAR) Trial cohort, and 18- and 36-month outcomes show continued compliance with therapy and effectiveness similar to 12 month outcomes.[16]

### SUMMARY

Conceptually, UAS via the hypoglossal nerve provides a mechanism to physiologically treat OSA using an implantable device. Basic science data support that UAS anatomically opens the airway and improves airflow. Strong prospective and randomized clinical data demonstrate long-term clinically significant improvements in objective sleep and respiratory outcomes over the duration of observation.

### REFERENCES

1. Isono S, Tanaka A, Nishino T. Dynamic interaction between the tongue and soft palate during obstructive apnea in anesthetized patients with sleep-disordered breathing. J Appl Physiol (1985) 2003;95:2257–64.

2. Remmers JE, deGroot WJ, Sauerland EK, et al. Pathogenesis of upper airway occlusion during sleep. J Appl Physiol (1985) 1978;44:931–8.
3. Mezzanotte WS, Tangel DJ, White DP. Influence of sleep onset on upper-airway muscle activity in apnea patients versus normal controls. Am J Respir Crit Care Med 1996;153:1880–7.
4. Patil SP, Schneider H, Marx JJ, et al. Neuromechanical control of upper airway patency during sleep. J Appl Physiol (1985) 2007;102:547–56.
5. McGinley BM, Schwartz AR, Schneider H, et al. Upper airway neuromuscular compensation during sleep is defective in obstructive sleep apnea. J Appl Physiol (1985) 2008;105:197–205.
6. Goding GS Jr, Eisele DW, Testerman R, et al. Relief of upper airway obstruction with hypoglossal nerve stimulation in the canine. Laryngoscope 1998;108:162–9.
7. Bellemare F, Pecchiari M, Bandini M, et al. Reversibility of airflow obstruction by hypoglossus nerve stimulation in anesthetized rabbits. Am J Respir Crit Care Med 2005;172:606–12.
8. Schwartz AR, Smith PL, Oliven A. Electrical stimulation of the hypoglossal nerve: a potential therapy. J Appl Physiol (1985) 2014;116:337–44.
9. Eisele DW, Smith PL, Alam DS, et al. Direct hypoglossal nerve stimulation in obstructive sleep apnea. Arch Otolaryngol Head Neck Surg 1997;123:57–61.
10. Eastwood PR, Barnes M, Walsh JH, et al. Treating obstructive sleep apnea with hypoglossal nerve stimulation. Sleep 2011;34(11):1479–86.
11. Goding GS Jr, Tesfayesus W, Kezirian EJ. Hypoglossal nerve stimulation and airway changes under fluoroscopy. Otolaryngol Head Neck Surg 2012;146:1017.
12. Kezirian EJ, Goding GS Jr, Malhotra A, et al. Hypoglossal nerve stimulation improves obstructive sleep apnea: 12-month outcomes. J Sleep Res 2014;23(1):77–83.
13. Van de Heyning PH, Badr MS, Baskin JZ, et al. Implanted upper airway stimulation device for obstructive sleep apnea. Laryngoscope 2012;122(7):1626–33.
14. Strollo PJ Jr, Soose RJ, Maurer JT, et al. Upper-airway stimulation for obstructive sleep apnea. N Engl J Med 2014;370(2):139–49.
15. Woodson BT, Gillespie MB, Soose RJ, et al. Randomized controlled withdrawal study of upper airway stimulation on USA: short- and long-term effect. Otolaryngol Head Neck Surg 2014;151(5):880–7.
16. Woodson BT, Soose RJ, Gillespie MB, et al. Three-year outcomes of cranial nerve stimulation for obstructive sleep apnea: The STAR trial. Otolaryngol Head Neck Surg 2016;154(1):181–8.

# Skeletal Surgery for Obstructive Sleep Apnea

José E. Barrera, MD[a,b,c],*

## KEYWORDS

- Obstructive sleep apnea • Surgery success • Surgery technique • Skeletal surgery
- Hyoid myotomy and suspension • Genioglossal advancement • Sliding genioplasty
- Maxillomandibular advancement

## KEY POINTS

- Combined with a uvulopalatopharyngoplasty, tongue-base surgeries, including the genioglossus advancement (GA), sliding genioplasty, and hyoid myotomy and suspension, have been developed to target hypopharyngeal obstruction.
- Total airway surgery consisting of maxillomandibular advancement with or without GA has shown significant success in patients with obstructive sleep apnea (OSA).
- Skeletal procedures for OSA with or without a palatal procedure is a proven technique for relieving airway obstruction during sleep.

## INTRODUCTION

Obstructive sleep apnea (OSA) continues to be a pervasive condition that is linked to an increased incidence of cardiovascular diseases, endocrine disorders, and overall increased health care utilization.[1] Multilevel surgery has been established as the mainstay of treatment for the surgical management of OSA. Skeletal surgery for OSA has traditionally consisted of a phased protocol to address airway obstruction secondary to nasopharyngeal, oropharyngeal, and hypopharyngeal obstruction. Combined with a uvulopalatopharyngoplasty (UPPP), tongue-base surgeries, including the genioglossus advancement (GA), sliding genioplasty (SG), and hyoid myotomy and suspension, have been developed to target hypopharyngeal obstruction. Total airway surgery, consisting of maxillomandibular advancement (MMA) with or without GA, has shown significant success in patients with OSA. Skeletal procedures for OSA with or without a palatal procedure are a proven technique for relieving airway obstruction during sleep.[2]

There are no commercial interests nor conflicts of interest associated with this publication. There is no funding for this work.
[a] Department of Surgery, Uniformed Services University, Bethesda, MD, USA; [b] Department of Otolaryngology, University of Texas Health Sciences Center, San Antonio, TX, USA; [c] Texas Facial Plastic Surgery and ENT, 14603 Huebner Road, Building 1, San Antonio, TX 78209, USA
* Texas Facial Plastic Surgery and ENT, 555 East Basse Road, Suite 201, San Antonio, TX 78209.
E-mail address: admin@drjosebarrera.com

Otolaryngol Clin N Am 49 (2016) 1433–1447
http://dx.doi.org/10.1016/j.otc.2016.07.006
0030-6665/16/© 2016 Elsevier Inc. All rights reserved.

It has been well established that skeletal advancement procedures typically accomplish a goal of 8 to 14 mm of advancement, thus increasing tension on the pharyngeal, genioglossus, and geniohyoid muscles with the goal of reducing the severity of sleep apnea.[1,3,4] Patients are traditionally selected for surgery based on the level of obstruction, which often occurs at the level of the base of tongue, although most patients demonstrate retropalatal obstruction as well. Since the introduction of a skeletal surgery to advance the genioglossus muscle along with UPPP, as described by Riley and colleagues,[1] multilevel reconstruction surgery has demonstrated improved outcomes in relieving OSA in those who demonstrate multilevel obstruction.[3,4]

Although physical examination, drug-induced sleep endoscopy (DISE), and polysomnography (PSG) help to guide the clinician's decision-making process in selecting patients who are candidates for GA, SG, or MMA combined with UPPP, intraoperative factors, such as length and width of the velum, degree of palatal and tongue-base obstruction, and concomitant lateral pharyngeal wall obstruction, are currently being studied. DISE[5,6] and sleep MRI[7,8] have emerged as modalities to diagnose the site of airway obstruction before surgery.

## Preoperative Considerations

All patients considered for skeletal surgery are first diagnosed by PSG, Epworth evaluation, and fiberoptic laryngoscopy. Candidates for surgery present with an apnea-hypopnea index (AHI) of more than 5 events per hour, and/or a respiratory disturbance index (RDI) greater than 5 with an Epworth Sleepiness Scale (ESS) greater than 8, who either did not tolerate, or refused a trial of continuous positive airway pressure (PAP). Presurgical patients present with evidence of obstruction as demonstrated by awake physical examination documenting Friedman II or III classification. Exclusion criteria for skeletal surgery include age younger than 12 years, chronic pulmonary disease on oxygen, and those affected with an untreated sleep disorder other than OSA that represents their primary sleep disorder. Preoperative assessment included history taking; ESS evaluation; complete physical examination; and PSG. Outcomes are defined by success, cure, and responder criteria. Success is defined as an AHI less than 20 and/or a 50% decrease in AHI of the preoperative value. Cure is defined as an AHI less than 5 events per hour. Responder is defined as significant improvement in the AHI and/or RDI after surgical intervention.

Obstruction can occur at a number of points in the airway. Physical examination of these patients may reveal hypertrophy of the adenoids and tonsils, retrognathia, micrognathia, macroglossia, deviation of the nasal septum, turbinate hypertrophy, a thick short neck, or tumors in the nasopharynx or hypopharynx. Both primary and secondary medical conditions are associated with OSA, owing to their effects on the upper airway anatomy. These may include temporomandibular joint disorders, myxedema, goiter, acromegaly, and lymphoma.

Fiberoptic nasopharyngoscopy is used to identify obstruction at the nasopharynx, oropharynx, and hypopharynx, and to rule out laryngeal anomalies. It can help estimate the degree of lateral wall collapse, palatal narrowing, and tongue-base obstruction. The site of obstruction can be classified by Fujita classification, with type I being palatal obstruction only, type II presenting as a combined palatal and tongue-base obstruction, and type III a tongue-base obstruction pattern only. Without performing fiberoptic evaluation, the site of obstruction may not be discernable.

Cephalometric evaluation is a simple way to evaluate individual patient upper airway site of obstruction. Cephalometric evaluation has long been used in evaluation of the airway in OSA. The metrics used for evaluation are SNA, SNB, PNS, Mandibular angle, posterior airway space (PAS), and MP-H (**Fig. 1**). These metrics are used to evaluate

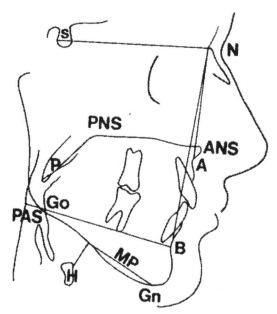

**Fig. 1.** Cephalometric figure. (*From* Riley RW, Powell NB, Guilleminault C. Inferior mandibular osteotomy and hyoid myotomy suspension for obstructive sleep apnea: a review of 55 patients. J Oral Maxillofac Surg 1989;47(2):160; with permission.)

preoperative obstruction and follow postoperative results. It is recommended that this 2-dimensional radiograph be supplemented with a 3-dimensional fiberoptic to evaluate the airway. At our institution, the most consistent finding is a narrowed PAS and low hyoid position (MP-H).[9]

The definitive objective test is a study during sleep. The gold standard at present is an attended PSG evaluation. This level I study assesses the cardiorespiratory system, revealing oxygenation information, and records electroencephalogram, electrooculogram, and electromyogram. It reveals sleep stage information and estimates the percentage of apnea, hypopneas, and respiratory-related events during sleep. Ambulatory studies are estimated as level III and do not determine sleep stage data.

### Surgical Technique

Retropalatal obstruction is addressed with UPPP. Fujita and colleagues[10] introduced UPPP with tonsillectomy in 1979. Many modifications have been published; the basic procedure involves palate shortening with closure mucosal incisions, tonsillectomy, and lateral pharyngoplasty. For multilevel surgery candidates, patients undergo a UPPP with GA or SG.

### Genioglossal Advancement

The GA must be distinguished from tongue suspension. The advancement of the geniotubercle in the GA procedure is distinct from suture fixation and suspension of the tongue base. The tongue suspension technique does not advance the mandible and is not considered a skeletal procedure. GA is performed as described by Riley and colleagues.[11] To review, after local anesthetic with a concentration of 1:100,000, epinephrine is injected at the lower gingivolabial sulcus, an incision is created along the anterior mandible. Subperiosteal dissection is then achieved exposing the anterior face of the mandible along its inferior border and then laterally identifying the mental neurovascular bundles. A horizontal window osteotomy is then created using a sagittal saw approximately 5 mm below the roots of the canine and approximately 10 mm above the inferior border of the mandible. The bone cut is then connected with 2 vertical osteotomies completing the rectangular window. Making a bicortical anterior osteotomy performs the GA. The width of the mandible, which had been pulled forward via the window osteotomy, is measured. The facial cortex and medullary bone is then removed and the lingual cortex holding the origin of the genioglossus muscle is rotated perpendicular to the window osteotomy. The osteotomized segment is then secured inferiorly with a single bicortical titanium screw (**Fig. 2**). Closure is performed with a 3 to 0 chromic with closure of the mentalis muscle and gingiva-buccal sulcus.

### Sliding Genioplasty Technique

The SG is an advancement genioplasty that is occasionally recommended for patients with microgenia due to both a retrognathic and foreshortened mandible. Patients in whom the GA cannot be performed due to increased risk for tooth injury or in patients with significant retrognathia greater than 2 cm from the subnasale vertical tangent may be considered for SG. The SG procedure seldom includes the

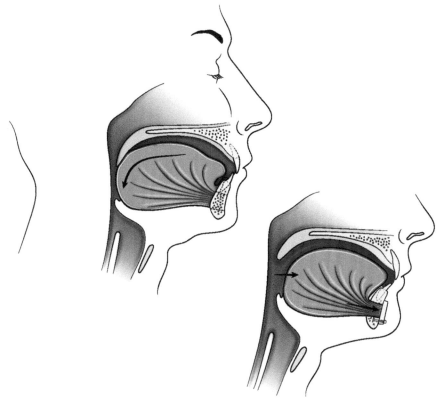

**Fig. 2.** GA. Anterior inferior osteotomy shown with 2.0-mm screw fixation. (*Courtesy of* Robert Jackler, MD, Stanford, CA.)

entire genial tubercle, thereby not affecting pull on the genioglossal muscle. It will likely pull the geniohyoid muscle that may lead to an unfavorable vector on the tongue base. The procedure may be amenable for patients with retro-epiglottic obstruction. The SG is performed through subperiosteal dissection with exposure of the inferior border of the anterior mandible. A reciprocating saw is used to cut both lateral edges of the parasymphysis along its inferior border and then laterally tapering the cut below the mental neurovascular bundles. The SG operation is often performed for both functional and aesthetic concerns. When the anterior osteotomy incorporates the geniotubercle through adjacent vertical window osteotomies, the operation is described as a mortised genioplasty. A patient with mild OSA with microgenia and nasal obstruction is depicted with postoperative cure in OSA after functional rhinoplasty and SG in **Fig. 3**.

### Hyoid Myotomy and Suspension

There are 2 generally accepted techniques in performing hyoid myotomy and suspension; the hyoid-mandibular and the hyoid-thyroid technique.[1,12,13] The author describes the hyoid-thyroid technique in this publication. The hyoid bone is a U-shaped bone suspended by the omohyoid, mylohyoid, and geniohyoid muscle; hyoepiglottic ligament; and accessory strap and laryngeal muscles. Its intimate connection with the tongue base and epiglottis makes it a viable technique for addressing hypopharyngeal obstruction. The hyoid-thyroid technique is performed through a cervical neck incision overlying the hyoid bone. Dissection is performed in a subplatysmal plane to expose the hyoid bone. Infrahyoid release of the strap muscles is performed using electrocautery medial to the greater cornu of the hyoid. Mobilization and suspension of the hyoid bone over the thyroid cartilage is performed using 2 to 0 Prolene sutures as depicted (**Fig. 4**). The hyoid-thyroid technique may be performed under local anesthesia with fiberoptic evaluation of the hypopharynx or under general anesthesia with concomitant GA, SG, or UPPP.

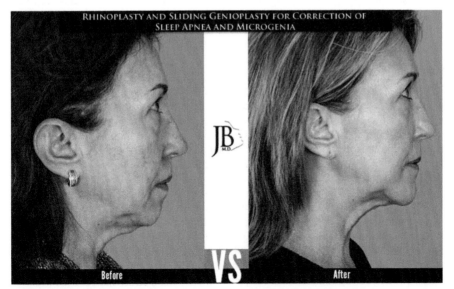

**Fig. 3.** SG patient with mild OSA (*left*: before; *right*: after functional rhinoplasty and SG).

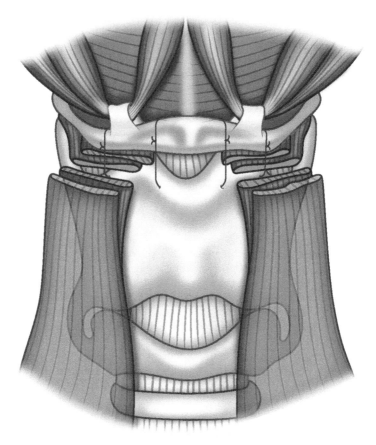

**Fig. 4.** Hyoid myotomy and suspension to thyroid cartilage technique. Conservative resection of the infrahyoid musculature is shown with suture suspension to the thyroid cartilage. (*Courtesy of* Robert Jackler, MD, Stanford, CA.)

### Maxillomandibular Advancement

Patients who have had incomplete response or failed to respond to phase I intervention may be considered for a phase II operation or MMA. In addition, patients with significant skeletal-dental deformity with OSA may be candidates for MMA. The MMA advances the midface and provides more room for the tongue. Additionally, the sagittal split osteotomy of the mandible places additional tension on the tongue-hyoid complex. Several publications have described the use of MMA in treating large series of patients with OSA.[14–19]

A bilateral sagittal ramus osteotomy is performed through a posterior gingivobuccal incision. Care is taken to identify the lingula of the mesial ascending ramus and the inferior alveolar nerve. A Hunsuck osteotomy is made with Lindeman burr or reciprocating blade (**Fig. 5**). The sagittal osteotomy then connects the ascending ramus cuts with the Dalpont osteotomy in the anterior mandible (**Fig. 6**). The ramus is then split with osteotomes. The amount of advancement is determined preoperatively from the orthognathic model surgery and/or virtual plan. Adjunctive orthodontic treatment is frequently necessary to obtain the desired occlusion and to eliminate

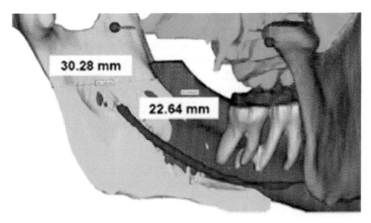

**Fig. 5.** MMA. Note Hunsuck osteotomy is made above the lingula. In this VSP, the width of the ramus at the osteotomy is 30.28 mm with the inferior alveolar nerve emanating 22.64 mm from the ramus. The inferior alveolar nerve is shown in red.

dental compensations that would otherwise limit the amount of advancement. Presurgical orthodontic evaluation with modeling may be considered before surgery but is not necessary. A thorough discussion is made with the patient to consider accompanying skeletal-dental abnormalities, and perioperative and postoperative management. Most patients retain their preoperative occlusion without need for orthodontic management. After advancement with the standard surgical technique, the fragments are rigidly fixed with screws or bone plates. For large advancements of 7 mm or more, long-term stability is enhanced with a 5-day to 7-day course of maxillomandibular fixation using orthodontic bands.

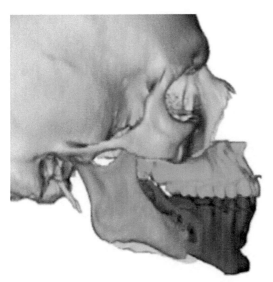

**Fig. 6.** MMA surgery depicting Lefort I osteotomy with bilateral sagittal split osteotomy with fixation is shown. Note sagittal split and anterior Dalpont osteotomy proposed and shown with advancement.

Combined advancement of the maxilla and mandible is the most recent and efficacious surgical procedure for the treatment of OSA. The surgical technique includes a standard Le Fort I osteotomy in combination with the aforementioned mandibular sagittal split osteotomy. A concomitant GA, as previously described, is an adjunct and recommended to improve tongue advancement (**Fig. 7**). MMA surgery may result in some facial change, which is most often favorable. However, the patient must be made aware of the possibility of any unfavorable aesthetic outcomes that may occur from this surgical procedure.

## MANDIBULAR SETBACK PROCEDURES

Mandibular setback procedures are composed of SG setbacks for a prominent chin in the aesthetic patients and bilateral sagittal split osteotomies performed for setback in the class III prognathic patients. In a small number of patients, a mandibular setback procedure can be the initiating factor in the development of OSA. Riley and colleagues[20] reported on 2 patients who developed OSA after mandibular setback surgery for correction of class III malocclusion and skeletal prognathism. Preoperative evaluation of these patients showed no symptoms of sleep apnea before surgery. Postoperatively, both patients began to snore loudly. PSG confirmed the presence of OSA syndrome. A comparative examination of the preoperative and postoperative lateral cephalograms of each patient showed a more inferiorly positioned hyoid bone and a narrowing of the pharyngeal airway. The report publication warns of the possibility of resultant OSA secondary to mandibular setback surgery, therefore caution should be heralded with this technique.

In an attempt to identify those patients potentially at risk for OSA, all patients who are planned for mandibular setback procedures should be questioned preoperatively and postoperatively about the presence or absence of snoring, excessive daytime

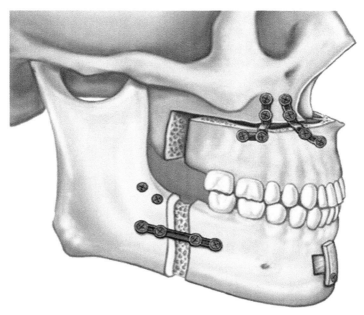

**Fig. 7.** MMA with GA. (*From* Barrera JE, Powell NB, Riley RW. Facial skeletal surgery in the management of adult obstructive sleep apnea syndrome. Clinics in Plastic Surgery 2007;34(3):565–73; with permission.)

sleepiness, or observed apneas during sleep. A PSG is recommended before consideration of mandibular setback procedures in these patients. Although the vast majority of patients who undergo mandibular setbacks are able to adapt to the changes in the skeletal and muscular apparatus, there is a subset of patients who may be at risk for developing overt signs of OSA.

## SURGICAL RESULTS
### Genioglossal Advancement

GA is a simple technique that does not move the teeth or jaw and therefore does not affect the dental bite. The GA is a procedure performed as a solitary hypopharyngeal procedure or in combination with MMA.[21] The technique places the genioglossus under tension and this tension may be sufficient to keep the base of tongue region open during sleep. This procedure does not gain more room for the tongue and thus must be considered a limited procedure that is dependent on the thickness of the individual's anterior mandible (mean thickness 12–18 mm). In addition, the existing laxity to the tongue during sleep is a factor on how much tension is gained when the genial tubercle is moved. In a flaccid tongue, the movement may all or partially be taken up by the advancement and little or no improvement may be attained. A paucity exists in determining the amount of tension needed or the critical distance the genial tubercle needs to move for effective posterior airway space improvement. An early study has determined that the tension-to-width ratio associated with geniotubercle advancement surgery may be an indicator for surgical response in patients with OSA.[22] These 2 factors limit our preoperative ability to accurately or consistently predict clinical outcomes. A meta-analysis evaluated success rates of genioglossal advancement to be between 39% and 78%.[23] Results of GA as a sole procedure for treatment of hypopharyngeal obstruction has been published in patients with severe OSA with success of more than 60% in 3 studies and oxyhemoglobin saturation results in 2 studies showing improvement in low oxyhemoglobin saturation (LSAT) in both studies. Only one study controlled for body mass index (BMI) and all 4 studies were level 4 Evidence based Medicine (EBM). The overall success rate was 62%. Our published clinical outcomes for success rates for GA with UPPP are 61%. Other centers have reported similar results with this procedure.

Complications associated with GA include tooth injury or loss, paresthesias, mandibular fracture, difficulty swallowing, wound infection, nonunion, and malunion of the mandible. Evaluation of swallow before and after GA has shown no increased incidence of swallow or speech dysfunction.[24]

### Sliding Genioplasty

SG is considered a surgical adjunctive procedure mostly used in orthognathic surgery and aesthetic chin augmentation surgery. The mortised genioplasty technique described, which incorporates the genioglossus with an SG, has been studied in patients with OSA. The overall success rate has been reported to be 48%. In this study, there were 2 factors contributing to success: (1) a low preoperative BMI, BMI less than 30, and (2) a preoperative AHI less than 50. If these factors were ascribed, the successful result of the operation was 64% and 71%, respectively, in these subsets of patients.[25]

### Genioglossal Advancement with Hyoid Myotomy

In 1989, Riley and colleagues[1,12] published a review of 55 patients with OSA who were treated with GA and hyoid myotomy with suspension (GAHM). Forty-two patients presented with type II Fujita classification showing obstruction at both the oropharynx and hypopharynx and received concomitant UPPP and GAHM. Six patients were determined to have obstruction localized to the base of the tongue (type III) and under-went GAHM only. Seven patients had failed previous UPPP and also underwent GAHM alone. All patients were reevaluated 6 months following surgery by PSG. Thirty-seven patients (67%) were considered to be responders to surgery based on the PSG results. GA ranged from 8 to 18 mm with a mean of 13 mm. All responders to surgery showed significant improvement in their RDI and oxygen desaturation events. Eighteen patients (33%) were considered nonresponders and failed to show significant improvement by PSG. The presence of preexisting chronic obstructive pul-monary disease was found to be a determining factor in increasing the risk of failure.

In 1994, Riley and colleagues[13] modified his technique for hyoid suspension by fixing the hyoid to the thyroid cartilage instead of the anterior margin of the mandible (see **Fig. 4**). When this modified technique was performed with inferior mandibular osteotomy, in lieu of the original hyoid suspension technique, the surgical response rate (with or without UPPP) was raised to 79.2%. The 5 nonresponders in this study of 24 patients achieved postoperative RDI values close to levels at which they would have been considered surgical responders.

A meta-analysis review of GAHM reveals an overall success rate of 55%. The pub-lished studies report a large cohort of obese patients with elevated AHI. Successful outcomes of 74% were associated with lower BMI, LSAT greater than 70, and AHI less than 60. A favorable SNB angle on cephalometric evaluation portended improved success rates.[23] Other investigators have reported that patients who have undergone GAHM have improved outcomes when presenting with normal pulmonary function, normal skeletal mandibular development, and the absence of obesity.[26] The most serious reported complication from a hyoid suspension has been severe aspiration in one patient, in which the thyrohyoid membrane was totally sectioned.[27] Other com-plications have included wound infections, transient sensory disturbances of the mental nerve, and mandibular fracture. An advantage to hyoid suspension is that it cir-cumvents the need for maxillomandibular fixation and does not affect the occlusion.[26,27]

### Hyoid Myotomy and Suspension

Success rates have varied in hyoid myotomy and suspension from 17% to 78% in 4 studies, all level 4 EBM.[23] However, these studies have been reported with associated UPPP or GA surgeries. In addition, the literature has not clearly delineated surgical re-sults by hyoid suspension technique.

A recent meta-analysis evaluated tongue suspension with UPPP, GA with UPPP, and GA with tongue suspension and hyoid-to-mandibular suspension. The results demonstrated success in 62.3%, 61.6%, and 61.1%, respectively. There was no significant difference between groups 2 and 3 compared with group 1. However, when tongue suspension was performed alone, the success rate dropped to 36.6%.[28]

### Maxillomandibular Advancement

Several investigators have described the use of MMA in treating large series of pa-tients with OSA.[14–19,29,30] In a series of 23 patients, Waite and colleagues[14] reported surgical success with MMA as 65% based on a postsurgical RDI of less than 10. Riley and colleagues[15] reported the largest series of patients with OSA treated with MMA in which 98% (89 of 91) were successfully treated based on a postoperative RDI of less than 20 with at least a 50% reduction in the RDI compared with the preoperative study. Hochban and colleagues[16] reported a 98% success rate on 38 patients with OSA consecutively treated with a 10-mm MMA as the primary surgery with postoperative

RDI less than 10 as the criteria to success. Prinsell[17] reported a 100% success rate based on a postoperative RDI of less than 15, an apnea index (AI) of less than 5, or a reduction in the RDI and AI of greater than 60% in patients who underwent MMA with and without GA. Lee and colleagues[18] proposed a 3-phased protocol for the surgical treatment of patients with OSA whereby phase I consisted of UPPP and GA or SG. If not successful, in phase 2, patients underwent MMA. A hyoid myotomy and suspension was reserved as a phase 3 surgery for failure. Phase 1 patients achieved success in 69% of cases (24 of 35 patients). Of the 11 stage 1 failures, 3 elected to proceed to phase 2 with MMA. All patients who underwent MMA had a postoperative RDI of less than 10, indicating a 100% response rate. No patient required hyoid myotomy and suspension. Bettega and colleagues[19] treated 51 consecutive patients with OSA, with 44 patients achieving a success rate of 22.7% (10 of 44) after UPPP and GAHM. Twenty patients underwent MMA as part of a phase 2 protocol. Of these, 75% (15 of 20) were considered to be surgical responders based on a postoperative RDI of less than 15 and at least a 50% reduction in the RDI. Of the 5 failures, 3 had postoperative RDIs of less than 20.

Riley and colleagues[29] describe MMA surgery as being a total airway surgery, having an effect on the posterior airway space (PAS) in the retropalatal and retrolingual space. PAS consistently increases with MMA. Caples and colleagues[30] published a meta-analysis comparing primary versus phased (secondary) MMA. In 234 patients receiving primary MMA, the mean preoperative AHI across all studies was 54.5 events per hour with resultant AHI of 7.7 events per hour postoperative. In 201 patients receiving secondary MMA, the mean preoperative AHI was 68.3 events per hour with 8.9 events per hour postoperatively. The mean BMI of patients with primary MMA was 29.1 compared with 36.6 in patients with secondary MMA. Holty and Guillenminault[31] published their meta-analysis reporting the clinical efficacy and safety of MMA surgery. Twenty-seven published articles reported on 320 patients with a mean AHI of 63.9 events per hour and a postoperative improvement of 9.5 events per hour postoperatively ($P>.001$). They reported that success was achieved with the greater degree of maxillary advancement. The major and minor complication rates were reported at 1.0% and 3.1%. Potential complications of MMA include surgical relapse, nonunion, bleeding, malocclusion, infection, unfavorable changes in facial appearance, and permanent or temporary sensory disturbances of the inferior alveolar and infraorbital nerves.[26] The long-term skeletal stability of MMA has been shown to be quite good. Louis and colleagues[32] showed a mean relapse of $0.9 \pm 1.8$ mm among 20 patients receiving maxillary advancement who underwent MMA for OSA with a mean follow-up period of 18.5 months (range 6–29 months). There was no statistical difference in the 3 groups based on advancement of 6 mm, 7 to 9 mm, and 10 mm or greater. Other reports have confirmed the stability of MMA surgery long term. Nimkarn and colleagues[33] showed that in 19 MMAs with SG patients that surgical stability was achieved over 1 year.[33]

MMA is considered the most efficacious procedure for expanding the pharyngeal airway and improving or eliminating OSA. It remains the best current alternative to tracheostomy.[26] Indications for this procedure include severe mandibular deficiency (SNB <74°), moderate to severe OSA (RDI >15, oxygen desaturations <90%), hypopharyngeal narrowing, and failure of other forms of treatment.[26] The success rate of MMA appears to increase when adjunctive procedures, such as UPPP, GA, lingual tonsillectomy and midline glossectomy, and nasal reconstruction, are considered in the phased treatment of patients with OSA.

Adjunctive orthodontic therapy may be considered in patients selected for MMA as long as airway protection by way of PAP therapy or an oral appliance as determined by

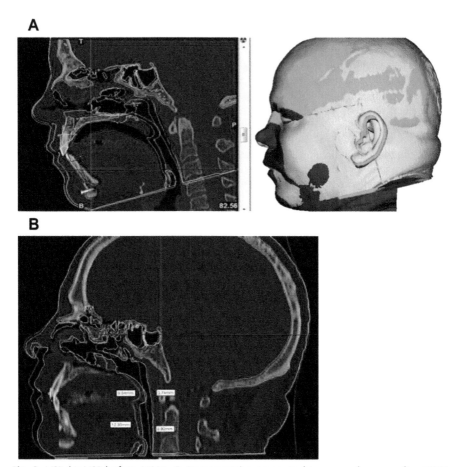

**Fig. 8.** VSP (*A*: VSP before MMA; *B*: Postoperative computed tomography scan after MMA surgery).

PSG is ensured. Presurgical orthodontics improves the postoperative occlusion and eliminates preexisting dental compensations that would otherwise limit the amount of advancement. Maximum advancement of the facial skeleton and maintenance of a functional occlusion and acceptable aesthetics are the goals of surgical-orthodontic correction.[26] The author reports his experience with integration of virtual surgical planning (VSP) and the treatment of OSA with MMA surgery. Although VSP has previously been reported for treating skeletal-dental abnormalities and dental implant surgery, a paucity of knowledge exists reporting the feasibility and resultant outcome measures when virtual surgical planning is used for planning maxillary and mandibular surgery for patients with OSA. A case series of 4 subjects with a mean RDI and AHI of 86.1 and 75.5 events per hour, respectively, and an LSAT of 73% underwent MMA either as a phased approach or as a single treatment. Postoperatively, the mean RDI and AHI improved to 4.53 and 2.70 events per hour, respectively ($P$<.008), with an LSAT of 87%. Significant improvement in the posterior airway space at the occlusal and mandibular planes were achieved, $P$<.05, and the tooth-to-lip measurement was preserved ($P$ = .92). VSP is a feasible tool used for predicting surgical outcome measures in MMA surgery for patients with OSA.[34]

## CASE STUDY

A 40-year-old man with severe OSA, notably an AHI of 70.9 events per hour, LSAT of 75%, RDI of 88.1, and ESS of 13 presented for surgical evaluation after PAP failure. His BMI was 29.3 kg/m². He underwent an uvulopalatal flap and geniotubercle advancement with a resultant improvement to AHI 13.3, LSAT 89% (<5 min), RDI 66.4, and ESS 12 with a BMI of 30.78. Due to his continued OSA and cognitive derangement, he underwent MMA surgery. VSP was performed to evaluate the patient and the patient underwent MMA based on the VSP.

His resultant PSG performed 17 months postoperative showed an AHI of 2.6 events per hour, LSAT 84% (<1 minute), and RDI of 3.7 with a BMI of 27.5 kg/m². The improvement in occlusal and mandibular airway measures were significant, 3.74 to 9.84 mm and 8.92 to 12.3 mm, respectively, $P<.05$. Tooth-to-lip measures were not significantly affected despite the achieved 8-mm advancement in the maxilla and mandible with 3-mm impaction, while the preoperative facial aesthetic profile was preserved (**Fig. 8**).

## SUMMARY

A multilevel and phased approach based on the patient's level of obstruction has increased sleep surgery's overall success in reducing the severity of OSA.[1–3] This logical, stepwise approach identifies patients who demonstrate retropalatal and/or hypopharyngeal obstruction. GA, SG, hyoid myotomy and suspension, and MMA address retrolingual obstruction, and may be used alone or in combination with other upper airway surgeries, most commonly UPPP. The goal of surgery is to improve airflow around the base of tongue and reduce the number of obstructive events that occur during sleep. MMA has reported the highest success and cure rates of all procedures but must be tailored to the appropriate patient.

## REFERENCES

1. Riley R, Guilleminault C, Powell N, et al. Mandibular osteotomy and hyoid bone advancement for obstructive sleep apnea: a case report. Sleep 1984;7(1):79–82.
2. Lewis MR, Ducic Y. Genioglossus muscle advancement with the genioglossus bone advancement technique for base of tongue obstruction. J Otolaryngol 2003;32(3):168–73.
3. Emara TA, Omara TA, Shouman WM. Modified genioglossus advancement and uvulopalatopharyngoplasty in patients with obstructive sleep apnea. Otolaryngol Head Neck Surg 2011;145(5):865–71.
4. Riley RW, Powell NB, Guilleminault C. Inferior sagittal osteotomy of the mandible with hyoid myotomy-suspension: a new procedure for obstructive sleep apnea. Otolaryngol Head Neck Surg 1986;94(5):589–93.
5. den Herder C, van Tinteren H, de Vries N. Sleep endoscopy versus Mallampati score in sleep apnea and scoring. Laryngoscope 2005;115:735–9.
6. Rodriguez-Bruno K, Goldberg AN, McCulloch CE, et al. Test-retest reliability of drug-induced sleep endoscopy. Otolaryngol Head Neck Surg 2009;140:646–51.
7. Barrera JE, Holbrook HS, Santos J, et al. Sleep MRI: novel technique to identify airway obstruction in obstructive sleep apnea. Otolaryngol Head Neck Surg 2009;140:423–5.
8. Barrera JE. Sleep magnetic resonance imaging: dynamic characteristics of the airway during sleep in obstructive sleep apnea. Laryngoscope 2011;121:1327–35.

9. Partinen M, Quera-Salva MA, Jamieson A, et al. Obstructive sleep apnea and cephalometric roentgenograms: the role of anatomic upper airway abnormalities in the definition of abnormal breathing during sleep. Chest 1988;93:1199–205.

10. Fujita S, Conway W, Zorick F, et al. Surgical correction of anatomic abnormalities in obstructive sleep apnea syndrome: uvulopalatopharyngoplasty. Otolaryngol Head Neck Surg 1981;89:923–34.

11. Riley RW, Powell NB, Guilleminault C. Maxillary, mandibular, and hyoid advancement for treatment of obstructive sleep apnea: a review of 40 patients. J Oral Maxillofac Surg 1990;48:20–6.

12. Riley RW, Powell NB, Guilleminault C. Inferior mandibular osteotomy and hyoid myotomy suspension for obstructive sleep apnea: a review of 55 patients. J Oral Maxillofac Surg 1989;47:159–64.

13. Riley RW, Powell NB, Guilleminault C. Obstructive sleep apnea and the hyoid: a revised surgical procedure. Otolaryngol Head Neck Surg 1994;111:717–21.

14. Waite PD, Wooten V, Lachner J, et al. Maxillomandibular advancement surgery in 23 patients with obstructive sleep apnea syndrome. J Oral Maxillofac Surg 1989; 47:1256–61.

15. Riley RW, Powell NB, Guilleminault C. Obstructive sleep apnea syndrome: a review of 306 consecutively treated surgical patients. Otolaryngol Head Neck Surg 1993;108:117–25.

16. Hochban W, Conradt R, Brandenburg U, et al. Surgical maxillofacial treatment of obstructive sleep apnea. Plast Reconstr Surg 1997;99:619–26 [discussion: 627–8].

17. Prinsell JR. Maxillomandibular advancement surgery in a site-specific treatment approach for obstructive sleep apnea in 50 consecutive patients. Chest 1999; 116:1519–29.

18. Lee NR, Givens CD Jr, Wilson J, et al. Staged surgical treatment of obstructive sleep apnea syndrome: a review of 35 patients. J Oral Maxillofac Surg 1999; 57:382–5.

19. Bettega G, Pepin JL, Veale D, et al. Obstructive sleep apnea syndrome fifty-one consecutive patients treated by maxillofacial surgery. Am J Respir Crit Care Med 2000;162:641–9.

20. Riley RW, Powell NB, Guilleminault C, et al. Obstructive sleep apnea syndrome following surgery for mandibular prognathism. J Oral Maxillofac Surg 1987;45: 450–2.

21. Barrera JE, Riley RW, Powell NB. Facial skeletal surgery in the management of adult obstructive sleep apnea syndrome. Clin Plast Surg 2007;34:565–73.

22. Andrews J, Barrera JE. Does tension matter? A study of tension in geniotubercle advancement surgery. Otolaryngol Head Neck Surg 2012;145(2 Suppl):P270.

23. Kezirian EJ, Goldberg AN. Hypopharyngeal surgery in obstructive sleep apnea: an evidence-based medicine review. Arch Otolaryngol Head Neck Surg 2006; 132:206–13.

24. Rohrer J, Eller R, Santillan PG, et al. Geniotubercle advancement with a uvulopalatal flap and its effect on swallow function in obstructive sleep apnea. Laryngoscope 2015;125:758–61.

25. Hendler BH, Costello BJ, Silverstein K, et al. A protocol for uvulaopalatpharyngoplasty, mortised genioplasty, and maxillomandibular advancement in patients with obstructive sleep apnea: an analysis of 40 cases. J Oral Maxillofac Surg 2001;59:892–9 [discussion: 898–9].

26. Tiner BD, Waite PD. Surgical and nonsurgical management of obstructive sleep apnea. In: Miloro M, Ghali GE, Larsen PE, et al, editors. Peterson's principles of oral maxillofacial surgery. 2nd edition. BC Becker; 2004. Chapter 63. p. 1536–46.
27. Dattilo DJ, Aynechi M. Modification of the anterior mandibular osteotomy for genioglossus advancement with hyoid suspension for obstructive sleep apnea. J Oral Maxillofac Surg 2007;65(9):1876–9.
28. Handler E, Hamans E, Goldberg AN, et al. Tongue suspension: an evidence base review and comparison to hypopharyngeal surgery in OSA. Laryngoscope 2014; 124:329–36.
29. Riley RW, Powell NB, Guilleminault C. Obstructive sleep apnea syndrome: a surgical protocol for dynamic upper airway reconstruction. J Oral Maxillofac Surg 1993;51:742–7 [discussion: 748–9].
30. Caples SM, Rowley JA, Prinsell JR, et al. Surgical modifications of the upper airway for obstructive sleep apnea in adults: a systematic review and meta-analysis. Sleep 2010;33(10):1396–407.
31. Holty JE, Guillenminault C. Maxillomandibular advancement for the treatment of obstructive sleep apnea: a systematic review and meta-analysis. Sleep Med Rev 2010;14(5):287–97.
32. Louis PJ, Waite PD, Austin RB. Long-term skeletal stability after rigid fixation of Le Fort I osteotomies with advancements. Int J Oral Maxillofac Surg 1993;22:82–6.
33. Nimkarn Y, Miles PG, Waite PD. Maxillomandibular advancement surgery in obstructive sleep apnea syndrome patients: long-term surgical stability. J Oral Maxillofac Surg 1995;53:1414–8 [discussion: 1418–9].
34. Barrera JE. Virtual surgical planning improves the predictability of surgical outcomes measures in obstructive sleep apnea surgery. Laryngoscope 2014;124: 1259–66.

# Pediatric Obstructive Sleep Apnea

Zarmina Ehsan, MD[a], Stacey L. Ishman, MD, MPH[a,b,c],*

## KEYWORDS

- Obstructive sleep apnea • Pediatric • Diagnosis • Management

## KEY POINTS

- History and physical examination are not sufficient to diagnose obstructive sleep apnea (OSA) in children. Overnight in-laboratory polysomnography remains the gold standard for OSA diagnosis.
- Adenotonsillectomy is first-line therapy for pediatric OSA. Medical treatment may be considered for children with mild primary or persistent OSA.
- Positive airway pressure is a treatment option for children who have persistent OSA after adenotonsillectomy or who are not surgical candidates. Poor tolerability and adherence limit its use.
- Lateral neck radiographs, awake nasopharyngoscopy, drug-induced sleep endoscopy, cine MRI, and computed tomography are modalities commonly used to assess sites of obstruction in children with OSA.
- Although evidence is limited, bony or soft tissue upper airway surgery for OSA is reasonable for children who fail medical management, especially for those with lingual tonsil hypertrophy or sleep-state–dependent laryngomalacia.

## INTRODUCTION

Obstructive sleep apnea (OSA) is a sleep-related breathing disorder characterized by prolonged partial upper airway obstruction (hypopnea) and/or complete upper airway

Disclosures: Nothing to disclose.
Funding Sources: None.
Conflict of Interest: None.
[a] Division of Pulmonary Medicine, Cincinnati Children's Hospital Medical Center, 3333 Burnet Avenue, MLC 2021, Cincinnati, OH 45229, USA; [b] Division of Pediatric Otolaryngology – Head & Neck Surgery, Cincinnati Children's Hospital Medical Center, 3333 Burnet Avenue, MLC 2018, Cincinnati, OH 45229, USA; [c] University of Cincinnati School of Medicine, Department of Otolaryngology – Head & Neck Surgery, 231 Albert Sabin Way, MSB 6503, Cincinnati, Ohio 45267-0528, USA
* Pediatric Otolaryngology–Head & Neck Surgery and Division of Pulmonary Medicine-Upper Airway Center, Cincinnati Children's Hospital Medical Center, 3333 Burnet Avenue, MLC 2018, Cincinnati OH 45229-2018.
E-mail address: stacey.ishman@cchmc.org

Otolaryngol Clin N Am 49 (2016) 1449–1464
http://dx.doi.org/10.1016/j.otc.2016.07.001
oto.theclinics.com

obstruction (apnea).[1] The most recent diagnostic criteria for pediatric OSA[2] require one of the following clinical findings: snoring, labored/obstructed breathing, or daytime consequences (sleepiness, hyperactivity), along with 1 or more polysomnography (PSG) findings. These PSG findings include (1) greater than or equal to 1 obstructive event (obstructive or mixed apnea, or obstructive hypopnea) per hour of sleep, or (2) obstructive hypoventilation manifested by peripheral arterial carbon dioxide ($P_aCO_2$) greater than 50 mm Hg for greater than 25% of sleep time, coupled with snoring, paradoxic thoracoabdominal movement, or flattening of the nasal airway pressure waveform (**Table 1**).

### Nature of the Problem (Epidemiology)

OSA is documented in 1% to 5%[3] of children. Numerous studies report that OSA is associated with decreased neurocognitive, behavioral, and quality-of-life scores, as well as increased systemic blood pressure,[4–8] increased pulmonary sequelae,[9] and increased health care use.[2,3] Moreover, children with OSA are more likely to have hypertension and metabolic syndrome as adults.[10] Both neuropsychological behavior and quality of life tend to normalize after airway obstruction has resolved.[11,12] Early identification can expedite treatment and prevent or reverse many of these negative health consequences.

Conditions associated with an increased prevalence of pediatric OSA[13] include:

- Male gender, especially in adolescents
- Black race
- Family history of OSA
- Prematurity
- Obesity
- Allergic rhinitis
- Down syndrome
- Prader-Willi syndrome
- Neuromuscular disorders
- Chiari malformations/myelomeningocele
- Craniofacial anomalies (eg, achondroplasia and Pierre Robin sequence)[14]

### ANATOMY/PATHOPHYSIOLOGY

The pathophysiology of OSA is complex and multifactorial with neurologic factors contributing to its development. Diminished electromyogram responsiveness of upper airway dilator muscles to negative pharyngeal pressure, decreased respiratory arousal thresholds, and high loop gain are all key physiologic factors that contribute

| Table 1 Rating scale: OSA severity classification in children | |
|---|---|
| **OSA Severity** | **PSG Criteria (AHI; events/h)** |
| No OSA | <1 |
| Mild | >1 to <5 |
| Moderate | >5 to <10 |
| Severe | >10 |

Abbreviation: AHI, apnea-hypopnea index.

to OSA.[15,16] In addition, the upper airway typically becomes compromised secondary to soft tissue and/or bony abnormalities, thus prompting an evaluation of the 5 anatomic sites where obstruction most frequently occurs: the nose and nasopharynx, the posterior oropharynx, the lateral pharyngeal walls, the hypopharynx (base of the tongue), and the supraglottic larynx.

Persistent nasal airway obstruction may result from a deviated nasal septum, enlarged nasal turbinates, or polypoid changes. An assessment for these findings as well as that of a high-arched hard palate is also warranted. Anterior-posterior narrowing and lateral wall collapse of the posterior oropharynx have also been shown to contribute to OSA,[17] as have base-of-tongue obstruction, lingual tonsil hypertrophy, and supraglottic collapse.[18]

### Diagnosis

#### Overnight in-laboratory polysomnography

Overnight, in-laboratory PSG is the gold standard for diagnosing OSA in children.[1,19] A single overnight PSG has:

- Good test-retest reliability and consistency
- No significant first-night effect[20]
- Specific OSA severity criteria, which are shown in **Table 1**
- A lack of consensus regarding the exact cutoff levels for OSA severity
- A lack of consensus regarding when to use pediatric versus adult criteria for the diagnosis of OSA in adolescents[21]

#### Overnight oximetry

In a cross-sectional study of 349 children (median age of 4.5 years), abnormal nocturnal pulse oximetry had a 97% positive predictive value (PPV) but a 47% negative predictive value (NPV) for detecting OSA compared with PSG. Therefore, a positive oximetry result is useful to establish a diagnosis of OSA, whereas a negative result cannot be used to rule out OSA.[22]

#### Nap and ambulatory polysomnography

Nap PSGs are abbreviated studies that are typically performed during the daytime. For diagnosing pediatric OSA, they are reported to have a:

- Sensitivity of 69% to 74%
- Specificity of 60% to 100%
- PPV of 77% to 100%
- NPV of 17% to 70% to 17%[23,24]

Nap PSG is not recommended for the definitive diagnosis of OSA by either the American Academy of Sleep Medicine or the American Academy of Pediatrics, because it can underestimate the presence or severity of OSA compared with in-laboratory nocturnal PSG.

Unattended full-montage home PSG has been reported to be adequate and feasible in school-aged children.[25] These studies tend to underestimate the incidence of obstructive hypopnea events as well as overall OSA severity. Studies using a limited number of recording channels, and without electroencephalogram recording, have been found to have conflicting results.

#### Other noninvasive diagnostic methods

A study of the use of home video recording for screening OSA in children showed that a 30-minute video had a sensitivity of 94% and a specificity of 68%.[26] Several sleep questionnaires are also available to screen for OSA; however, validation studies comparing these with PSG data are scarce.[27–29] An in-depth review of available questionnaires was not able to identify any one tool with a sufficient combination of sensitivity and specificity.[30] Therefore, these tests are not considered standard of care in the evaluation of pediatric OSA.

## EVALUATION
### History and Physical Examination

Evaluation of children with OSA should include the common history and physical examination elements listed in **Box 1**. This evaluation often also includes awake flexible nasopharyngoscopy and laryngoscopy in the office to assess for nasal disorder, adenoidal hypertrophy, lingual tonsil hypertrophy, laryngomalacia, or other obstructing airway lesions. Although this evaluation is important, history and physical examination alone are rarely sufficient to diagnose OSA. Prolonged wait times and poor availability of pediatric sleep laboratories for overnight PSG have prompted a search for alternative diagnostic screening tools. These tools typically include a combination of history and physical examination findings,[31] but none have been found to be sufficient to predict OSA.[32]

### Imaging

Modalities used to evaluate children with OSA include:

- Lateral neck films to assess adenoidal size, nasal abnormalities, and lingual tonsil hypertrophy[33,34]

---

**Box 1**
**Symptom criteria and examination findings**

*History*

- Frequent snoring ($\geq$3 nights/wk)
- Labored breathing during sleep
- Gasps/snorting noises/observed episodes of apnea
- Sleep enuresis (especially secondary enuresis)
- Sleeping in a seated position or with the neck hyperextended
- Cyanosis
- Headaches on awakening
- Daytime sleepiness
- Attention-deficit/hyperactivity disorder
- Learning problems

*Physical examination*

- Underweight or overweight
- Tonsillar hypertrophy
- Adenoidal facies
- Micrognathia/retrognathia
- High-arched palate
- Failure to thrive
- Hypertension

---

- Cephalometric imaging, which may correlate with endoscopic findings[35]
- Cine MRI (described later in this article)
- Facial computed tomography (CT) for children with craniofacial disorders and bony abnormalities of the facial skeleton
- Videofluoroscopy and dynamic cine CT scans are less commonly used because of concerns regarding radiation exposure[36]

## Drug-induced Sleep Endoscopy

Drug-induced Sleep Endoscopy (DISE)
- Is used to identify sites of upper airway obstruction in adults and children with persistent OSA[20,37] **(Table 2)**[18]
- Was developed because sites of obstruction detected in awake patients do not always correlate with the sites of obstruction observed during sleep[38]
- Is useful to detect sleep state–dependent (late-onset) laryngomalacia[39]

The choice of anesthetic agent used during the evaluation is important given that these agents can alter airway dynamics and potentially influence examination findings.[40]

**Table 2**
**Summary of studies on DISE to identify site of obstruction for children with persistent OSA following adenotonsillectomy**

| Author | N | Mean Age (y) | Persistent OSA (%) | ID Site of Obstruction (%) | Comments |
|--------|---|--------------|--------------------|-----------------------------|----------|
| Myatt | 8 | NR | NR | 100 | Also recommend rigid bronchoscopy |
| Lin | 26 | 11 | 100 | NR | 61% postoperative AHI <5 |
| Chan, 2012 | 22 | 7 | NR | NR | For laryngomalacia Tx = supraglottoplasty |
| Digoy | 36 | NR | 100 | 100 | For sleep state–dependent laryngomalacia |
| Durr | 13 | 8 | 69 | 100 | Multilevel disease was common |
| Fung | 23 | 7 | NR | 100 | DS with more lingual and pharyngeal collapse |
| Truong | 39 | NR | 100 | NR | Effective ID collapse in persistent and primary OSA |
| Fishman | 28 | 8 | 100 | NR | ID more obstruction than awake endoscopy |
| Ulualp, & Szmuk,[41] 2013 | 82 | 6 | 100 | NR | Most with multilevel obstruction |
| Chan, 2014 | 23 | 2 | NR | NR | Evaluating 4-point grading scale |
| Wootten & Shott,[78] 2010 | 11 | 8 | 100 | NR | 92% had subjective improvement |

*Abbreviations:* DS, Down syndrome; ID, identify; N, total number of patients; NR, not reported; Tx, treatment.
*Adapted from* Manickam PV, Shott SR, Boss EF, et al. Systematic review of site of obstruction identification and non-CPAP treatment options for children with persistent pediatric obstructive sleep apnea. Laryngoscope 2015;126(2):495; with permission.

A recent systematic review on sites of obstruction[18] reported that:
- The most common location for single-site obstruction was the oropharyngeal lateral walls
- The most common locations for multiple-site obstruction were the oropharyngeal lateral walls and the velum

An evaluation of children before adenotonsillectomy showed that these children had complete airway obstruction; even those with only grade I and grade II tonsils.[41] Literature regarding how these modalities correlate with outcomes is scarce.[18] Several scoring systems have been described, but a uniform grading system for DISE findings has yet to be agreed on.

### Cine MRI

Cine MRI (**Table 3**)[18]
- Provides a high-resolution dynamic examination of the airway to identify sites of upper airway obstruction
- Has no radiation exposure
- Is particularly helpful when evaluating children with multiple sites of obstruction and to simultaneously identify primary and secondary sites of obstruction[42]
- Is performed with mild sedation using medications that most closely mimic natural sleep[43]
- Has been reported to identify the site of obstruction in 93% of cases[18]

### Management of pediatric obstructive sleep apnea
**Weight loss** In adults, a recent systematic review reported that both surgical and nonsurgical weight loss significantly improved OSA by reducing both the body mass index (BMI) and the apnea-hypopnea index (AHI).[44] Although the literature regarding weight loss for OSA in children is limited, research suggests that weight loss should be recommended in obese children with OSA.[45] Bariatric surgery is reserved for children failing medical weight loss, particularly those with significant comorbid medical conditions. The American Society for Metabolic and Bariatric

---

**Table 3**
**Summary of studies on cine MRI to identify site of obstruction for children with persistent OSA following adenotonsillectomy**

| Author | N | Mean Age (y) | Persistent OSA (%) | ID Site of Obstruction (%) | Comments |
|---|---|---|---|---|---|
| Shott & Donnelly,[42] 2004 | 15 | 10 | 100 | 93 | |
| Connelly et al | 27 | 10 | 100 | NR | ID obstructive sites in children with DS |
| Fricke et al | 89 | 10 | 58 | 33 | LTH only |

*Abbreviation:* LTH, lingual tonsillar hypertrophy.
*Adapted from* Manickam PV, Shott SR, Boss EF, et al. Systematic review of site of obstruction identification and non-CPAP treatment options for children with persistent pediatric obstructive sleep apnea. Laryngoscope 2015;126(2):493; with permission.

Surgery recommends that this approach be considered only for carefully selected, extremely obese adolescents meeting certain surgical criteria.[46] A small study of 10 children reported significant improvement in OSA severity after bariatric surgery; BMI decreased from a mean of 60.8 kg/m$^2$ (standard deviation [SD] $\pm$ 11.07 kg/m$^2$) to 41.6 kg/m$^2$ (SD $\pm$ 9.5 kg/m$^2$), whereas AHI decreased from 9.1 to 0.65 events per hour.[47]

**Medication** Montelukast and intranasal corticosteroids are both used to treat mild to moderate OSA in children. In a prospective double-blind randomized trial of 46 children, a 12-week treatment with daily oral montelukast reduced OSA severity by a few events per hour and reduced adenoidal hypertrophy.[48] In a large retrospective cohort study of more than 700 children with mild OSA who were treated with a combination of intranasal corticosteroids and oral montelukast for 12 weeks, the success rate of therapy was 81%. Follow-up PSG in 445 children revealed normalization of sleep parameters in 62% of children. The remaining 17% failed to show improvement or had worsening of their OSA. The investigators reported that nonresponders were more likely to be more than 7 years old and obese (BMI z-score >1.65).[49] Long-term studies to guide the duration of therapy and predict response are lacking.

**Positive airway pressure** Positive airway pressure (PAP) is positive pressure delivered via a nasal or full-face mask connected to a mechanical device that stents the airway by delivering intraluminal pressure that is higher than atmospheric pressure. PAP has been shown to effectively reduce the AHI and improve both subjective and objective sleep outcomes.[50] Continuous PAP (CPAP) is typically titrated in a sleep laboratory in order to determine the optimum pressure requirement to eliminate obstructive events by each patient.[51] A large series reported that the respiratory disturbance index (RDI) was reduced and oxygen saturation was increased in children aged 2 to 16 years using CPAP for OSA; however, at least 30% stopped the use of CPAP within 6 months.[52] Many children discontinue the use of CPAP because of the discomfort of the mask or the noise created by the device.[53] In addition, there are concerns that long-term use of the PAP mask can lead to skin defects or potentially facial flattening.[54]

Adherence to PAP therapy can be objectively measured with compliance downloads that are available on all commercially available machines in the United States.

**Oral appliances, orthodontics, and rapid maxillary expansion** Malocclusion and maxillofacial abnormalities have been associated with pediatric OSA.[55,56] Oral appliances are typically recommended for the treatment of mild to moderate OSA in children who have permanent dentition in place.[57] The use of oral appliances can also improve the tolerability of CPAP.[58] As with masks used for CPAP, oral appliances can result in craniofacial abnormalities caused by the prolonged mechanical forces exerted on the maxilla and mandible.

Rapid maxillary expansion (RME) has also been advocated to improve nasal patency while improving OSA severity and sleep quality.[59,60] These devices mechanically widen the palate and the nasal fossa. A study of a 60 children managed with RME reported a decrease in the mean AHI from 16.3 $\pm$ 2.5 to 8.3 $\pm$ 2.3 events/h at 4 weeks and 0.8 $\pm$ 1.3 events/h at 4 months posttreatment; the greatest benefit was achieved for children with mild to moderate OSA (AHI $\leq$15).[56] Other studies have shown incomplete response to RME.[61,62]

Evidence regarding orthodontic treatment of OSA in children is inconclusive. Therefore, conclusions regarding the treatment effect across multiple studies cannot be made.[63]

### Surgical management

Several surgical management options are available for children with OSA. Although adenotonsillectomy is primary therapy, several options exist for children who have persistent OSA after adenotonsillectomy (**Fig. 1**).

**Adenotonsillectomy and partial tonsillectomy** Practice guidelines from the AAP[19] and American Academy of Otolaryngology – Head and Neck Surgery (AAO-HNS)[64] both recommend adenotonsillectomy as primary therapy for OSA in healthy children older than age 2 years. Adenotonsillectomy has been reported to reduce daytime OSA symptoms and improve secondary outcomes of behavior, quality of life, and PSG findings, even in children who are not complete responders.[65]

A systematic review of cure rates reported that 34% of children had an RDI greater than or equal to 5 after surgery.[66] The investigators also reported significant differences in the resolution rates of OSA in uncomplicated children (74%) versus children with comorbidities (39%) (eg, morbid obesity, severe OSA, and younger than age 3 years). A meta-analysis of 4 studies and 110 obese children found that 51% had an AHI greater than 5 events/h after adenotonsillectomy.[67]

Partial tonsillectomy has been advocated for treatment of OSA because of the lower rates of bleeding and pain than are experience with complete tonsillectomy. However, partial tonsil removal carries a risk of tonsillar regrowth of between 0.5% to 17% and requires that children be monitored for recurrent OSA signs and symptoms.[68] Time to reevaluation for tonsil regrowth ranged from 1 to 18 months in the study that reported the highest regrowth rate (17%) with a mean of 1.2 years in the study with the lowest rate (0.5%).[68] A 4-year study of 375 children with yearly evaluations reported regrowth in 7.2% of children; 20 of the 375 subsequently underwent completion tonsillectomy.[68]

**Adenoidectomy** Although adenoidectomy is commonly used to treat OSA in young children or those without tonsillar hypertrophy, there are no level 1 studies of the

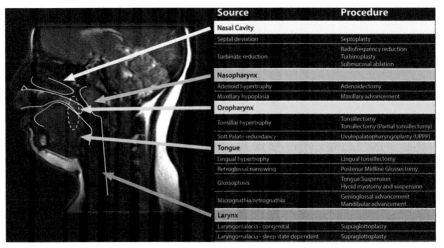

**Fig. 1.** Surgeries considered for children with persistent OSA after adenotonsillectomy by level of obstruction.

efficacy of adenoidectomy for the treatment of OSA. Regrowth of the adenoids and recurrence of OSA can necessitate revision adenoidectomy or adenotonsillectomy, particularly in children undergoing adenoidectomy before 6 years of age.[69]

**Nasal surgery** Nasal obstruction may result from a deviated nasal septum, nasal polyposis, choanal stenosis or atresia, or enlarged nasal turbinates. Although nasal obstruction is only infrequently the primary cause of OSA, it does contribute to OSA; treatment of this problem in affected children may therefore be helpful. A recent adult meta-analysis found that treatment of nasal obstruction can result in a reduction of the AHI by 11 events/h.[70] Pediatric studies focused on nasal treatment of OSA are scarce; however, a study combining adenotonsillectomy and inferior turbinate reduction showed improved OSA resolution compared with adenotonsillectomy alone.[71]

**Uvulopalatopharyngoplasty** Uvulopalatopharyngoplasty (UPPP) has been used for OSA treatment in adults with reported success rates ranging from 40% to 80%.[72] Higher success is seen in patients with large tonsils (3+ or 4+) and easy view of the uvula (modified Mallampati score 1 or 2).[73] Published articles reporting the usefulness and success of UPPP in children are limited to case series.[18] In children prone to hypernasality (eg, those with submucous clefts or Down syndrome), a more conservative excision of the soft palate may decrease rates of postoperative velopharyngeal insufficiency.[74]

For children with oropharyngeal lateral wall collapse, the expansion sphincter pharyngoplasty, as described by Pang and Woodson,[17] should also be considered.

**Lingual tonsillectomy** Enlarged lingual tonsils are a common site of residual obstruction in children with persistent OSA after adenotonsillectomy, especially for children with Down syndrome.[75] A systematic review of reported lingual tonsillectomy success rates showed a range from 57% to 88%, with higher failure rates in children with obesity, hypotonia, or craniofacial abnormalities (**Table 4**).[18] The technique has been described using several different surgical tools; however, coblation is presently the most commonly used technique.

**Base-of-tongue surgery** The aim of tongue-base procedures (see **Fig. 1**) is to decrease the amount of lingual tonsil or tongue-base tissue or prevent glossoptosis during sleep; the most commonly used techniques include lingual tonsillectomy,

**Table 4**
**Summary of lingual tonsillectomy studies for children with OSA**

| Author | N | Mean Age (y) | Resolution of OSA (%) | O₂ Sat Before/After Surgery (%) | AHI Before/After Surgery |
|---|---|---|---|---|---|
| Abdul-Aziz | 16 | NR | 68 | 84/91 | 10.5/3.2 |
| Chen | 68 | 11 | 57 | 89/91 | 11.8/5.7 |
| Truong | 31 | 7 | NR | NR | 18.3/9.7 |
| Lin | 26 | 11 | 61 | 89/90 | 14.7/8.1 |
| Wootten & Shott,[78] 2010 | 9 | 9 | 66 | 83/84 | 8.5/4.1 |

*Abbreviation:* O₂ Sat, oxygen saturation.

*Adapted from* Manickam PV, Shott SR, Boss EF, et al. Systematic review of site of obstruction identification and non-CPAP treatment options for children with persistent pediatric obstructive sleep apnea. Laryngoscope 2015;126(2):498; with permission.

posterior midline glossectomy, hyoid suspension, and tongue suspension. With the exception of lingual tonsillectomy, the efficacy of most of these procedures is better documented in the adult literature.

Posterior midline glossectomy is typically performed by making a midline wedge resection, with or without previous ultrasonography mapping of the lingual arteries, either open or submucosally. Although the coblator is the most commonly used instrument, the microdebrider, cautery, and other techniques may be used. In adults, a reduction in AHI by 50% has been reported with the use of midline posterior glossectomy.[76] Clark and colleagues[77] presented their experience with 22 patients undergoing posterior midline glossectomy, reporting a resolution rate of 59%.

Tongue-base suspension is a minimally invasive technique that provides a supporting sling to the tongue base as a treatment of glossoptosis.[78] Only 1 study has reported its used in children. This study reported a success rate of 61% (58% in children with Down syndrome) in 31 children when combined with radiofrequency to the base of tongue.[18]

Hyoid suspension is performed for children with a retroverted epiglottis to open up the posterior airway space and prevent glossoptosis during sleep. The hyoid bone may be stabilized to the thyroid cartilage or the mandible. In adults, this procedure has a success rate of 40% to 53% when performed as a solo procedure. There are no series reporting the use of this technique in children, although the senior author (SLI) uses this procedure for children older than age 5 years.

Traditional genioglossus advancement is performed with a midline segmental osteotomy technique. Bone cuts are made through the anterior mandible to create a full-thickness segment attached to the genioglossus muscle; this is advanced anteriorly and secured to the mandible, thus applying anterior traction to the genioglossus muscle. Clinical results in children have not been reported, and this surgery can only be performed in older children in whom secondary teeth have already erupted.

**Supraglottoplasty** Supraglottoplasty is the second most commonly reported procedure performed for persistent OSA.[18] This procedure is recommended for infants with laryngomalacia and OSA and for older children with sleep state–dependent (occult) laryngomalacia. A systematic review of supraglottoplasty reported success rates ranging from 58% to 72% (**Table 5**).[18]

**Other surgical options** Several additional surgical options exist. These options include mandibular and/or maxillary advancement surgery for children with significant craniofacial anomalies, tracheostomy for children with severe OSA and significant

| Table 5 | | | | | |
| --- | --- | --- | --- | --- | --- |
| **Summary of supraglottoplasty studies for children with OSA** | | | | | |
| Author | N | Mean Age (y) | Resolution of OSA (%) | O$_2$ Sat Before/ After Surgery (%) | AHI Before/ After Surgery |
| Chan | 24 | 7.3 | 58 | 88.0/88.8 (mean) | 14.9/4.9 |
| Chan & Truong | 9 | NR | NR | NR | 10.4/2.9 |
| Truong | 4 | NR | NR | NR | 9.7/5.7 |
| Digoy | 36 | NR | 72 | 83/86.5 | 13.3/4.1 |

*Adapted from* Manickam PV, Shott SR, Boss EF, et al. Systematic review of site of obstruction identification and non-CPAP treatment options for children with persistent pediatric obstructive sleep apnea. Laryngoscope 2015;126(2):497; with permission.

medical comorbidities, and infants without surgically identifiable obstruction or neurologic impairment.

### Multilevel Surgery

Multilevel surgery is the performance of surgery to address multiple sites of obstruction. This surgery can be performed concurrently or sequentially. Thus far, studies of multilevel surgery have predominantly been reported in adults. These studies have reported success rates of 50% to 60% for resolution of moderate to severe OSA. Although resolution of OSA is not always achieved, these surgeries have been reported to reduce the severity of OSA, thus allowing lower CPAP pressures. One pediatric study of 48 children who underwent multilevel surgery reported an 8.2% incidence of oropharyngeal scarring and stenosis when this surgery included lingual tonsillectomy and concurrent palate surgery.[79] Therefore, caution is recommended in these cases.

## PERIOPERATIVE MANAGEMENT

The preoperative evaluation of any child with OSA should include an investigation regarding a personal or family history of bleeding disorders, or problems experienced with anesthesia. If a bleeding risk is suspected, a more significant hematologic workup should be performed. In a recent study of children presenting with posttonsillectomy bleeding, 19% presented with abnormally increased prothrombin time, partial thromboplastin time, or platelet function assays, and 4% were diagnosed with a coagulopathy.[80] For children with long-term severe OSA, preoperative cardiac evaluation with an electrocardiogram or echocardiogram should be considered.

Because of the increased risk of anesthetic complications in children with OSA, the AAO-HNS advocates detailed communication between the surgeon and anesthesiologist regarding the severity of OSA and PSG findings before surgery,[81] to assist with appropriate intraoperative decision making.[81]

Children with OSA should be closely monitored postoperatively for hypoxemia and hypercarbia, because they are at greater risk for complications compared with healthy children. Because of an increased risk of perioperative complications, postoperative admission and observation are recommended for children in the following groups: age younger than 3 years, severe OSA, cardiac complications of OSA, failure to thrive, obesity, prematurity, recent respiratory infection, neuromuscular or craniofacial disorders, Down syndrome, mucopolysaccharidoses, and sickle cell disease.[19,64]

Children should receive adequate pain control, either with acetaminophen, ibuprofen, or narcotics. Studies suggest that children with OSA are more sensitive to the respiratory depressant effects of opioids and that these should thus be used judiciously.[82] In addition, in view of genetic variations in the metabolism of codeine, the US Food and Drug Administration has issued a warning against its use for children after adenotonsillectomy.[83]

## SUMMARY

- Screening for OSA is imperative in children with signs and symptoms of OSA, especially if surgery is being considered.
- Children with severe craniofacial anomalies have a high incidence of OSA and should be screened even if asymptomatic.[84]
- Awake flexible laryngoscopy, cine MRI, and DISE are all useful tools for assessing sites of obstruction and planning surgical interventions.

- Awake flexible laryngoscopy does not take into account the collapsibility of the airway that occurs with muscle relaxation during sleep, whereas DISE may be associated with false-positives resulting from excess muscle relaxation during anesthesia.
- For children with persistent OSA, medication, weight loss, PAP, oral appliance therapy, or surgery may all be options.
- Intranasal steroids and montelukast are beneficial in the resolution of mild OSA.
- RME can be considered in children with malocclusion and a high-arched palate.
- Palatine and lingual tonsil size, adenoid size, and the presence of laryngomalacia should be evaluated in children with persistent pediatric OSA.
- Lingual tonsillectomy and supraglottoplasty are the most common procedures reported for children with persistent OSA.
- Nasal surgery, UPPP, expansion pharyngoplasty, base-of-tongue surgery, craniofacial surgery, and tracheostomy can be used to treat persistent OSA.
- Outcomes research is needed to determine which patients are best treated with each treatment modality.

## REFERENCES

1. Loughlin GM, Brouillette RT, Brooke LJ, et al. Standards and indications for cardiopulmonary sleep studies in children (vol 153, pg 866, 1995). Am J Respir Crit Care Med 1996;153(6):U54.
2. Sateia MJ. International classification of sleep disorders-third edition: highlights and modifications. Chest 2014;146(5):1387–94.
3. Bixler EO, Vgontzas AN, Lin HM, et al. Sleep disordered breathing in children in a general population sample: prevalence and risk factors. Sleep 2009;32(6):731–6.
4. Enright PL, Goodwin JL, Sherrill DL, et al. Blood pressure elevation associated with sleep-related breathing disorder in a community sample of white and Hispanic children: The Tucson Children's Assessment of Sleep Apnea Study. Arch Pediatr Adolesc Med 2003;157(9):901–4.
5. Kohyama J, Ohinata JS, Hasegawa T. Blood pressure in sleep disordered breathing. Arch Dis Child 2003;88(2):139–42.
6. Leung LC, Ng DK, Lau MW, et al. Twenty-four-hour ambulatory BP in snoring children with obstructive sleep apnea syndrome. Chest 2006;130(4):1009–17.
7. Li AM, Au CT, Sung RYT, et al. Ambulatory blood pressure in children with obstructive sleep apnoea: a community based study. Thorax 2008;63(9):803–9.
8. Marcus CL, Greene MG, Carroll JL. Blood pressure in children with obstructive sleep apnea. Am J Respir Crit Care Med 1998;157(4 Pt 1):1098–103.
9. Mitchell RB. Sleep-disordered breathing in children: are we underestimating the problem? Eur Respir J 2005;25(2):216–7.
10. Sun SS, Grave GD, Siervogel RM, et al. Systolic blood pressure in childhood predicts hypertension and metabolic syndrome later in life. Pediatrics 2007;119(2):237–46.
11. Stewart MG, Glaze DG, Friedman EM, et al. Quality of life and sleep study findings after adenotonsillectomy in children with obstructive sleep apnea. Arch Otolaryngol Head Neck Surg 2005;131(4):308–14.
12. Tran KD, Nguyen CD, Weedon J, et al. Child behavior and quality of life in pediatric obstructive sleep apnea. Arch Otolaryngol Head Neck Surg 2005;131(1):52–7.
13. Marcus CL, Brooks LJ, Draper KA, et al. Diagnosis and management of childhood obstructive sleep apnea syndrome. Pediatrics 2012;130(3):e714–55.

14. Aurora RN, Zak RS, Karippot A, et al. Practice parameters for the respiratory indications for polysomnography in children. Sleep 2011;34(3):379–88.
15. Eckert DJ, White DP, Jordan AS, et al. Defining phenotypic causes of obstructive sleep apnea. Identification of novel therapeutic targets. Am J Respir Crit Care Med 2013;188(8):996–1004.
16. Marcus CL, McColley SA, Carroll JL, et al. Upper airway collapsibility in children with obstructive sleep apnea syndrome. J Appl Phys 1994;77(2):918–24.
17. Pang KP, Woodson BT. Expansion sphincter pharyngoplasty: a new technique for the treatment of obstructive sleep apnea. Otolaryngol Head Neck Surg 2007; 137(1):110–4.
18. Manickam PV, Shott SR, Boss EF, et al. Systematic review of site of obstruction identification and non-CPAP treatment options for children with persistent pediatric obstructive sleep apnea. Laryngoscope 2016;126(2):491–500.
19. Section on Pediatric Pulmonology, Subcommittee on Obstructive Sleep Apnea Syndrome. Clinical practice guideline: diagnosis and management of childhood obstructive sleep apnea syndrome. Pediatrics 2002;109(4):704–12.
20. Galluzzi F, Pignataro L, Gaini RM, et al. Drug induced sleep endoscopy in the decision-making process of children with obstructive sleep apnea. Sleep Med 2015;16(3):331–5.
21. Accardo JA, Shults J, Leonard MB, et al. Differences in overnight polysomnography scores using the adult and pediatric criteria for respiratory events in adolescents. Sleep 2010;33(10):1333–9.
22. Brouillette RT, Morielli A, Leimanis A, et al. Nocturnal pulse oximetry as an abbreviated testing modality for pediatric obstructive sleep apnea. Pediatrics 2000; 105(2):405–12.
23. Marcus CL, Keens TG, Ward SLD. Comparison of nap and overnight polysomnography in children. Pediatr Pulmonol 1992;13(1):16–21.
24. Saeed MM, Keens TG, Stabile MW, et al. Should children with suspected obstructive sleep apnea syndrome and normal nap sleep studies have overnight sleep studies? Chest 2000;118(2):360–5.
25. Tan HL, Kheirandish-Gozal L, Gozal D. Pediatric home sleep apnea testing: slowly getting there! Chest 2015;148(6):1382–95.
26. Sivan Y, Kornecki A, Schonfeld T. Screening obstructive sleep apnoea syndrome by home videotape recording in children. Eur Respir J 1996;9(10):2127–31.
27. Chervin RD, Weatherly RA, Garetz SL, et al. Pediatric sleep questionnaire: prediction of sleep apnea and outcomes. Arch Otolaryngol 2007;133(3):216–22.
28. Constantin E, Tewfik TL, Brouillette RT. Can the OSA-18 quality-of-life questionnaire detect obstructive sleep apnea in children? Pediatrics 2010;125(1):E162–8.
29. Borgstrom A, Nerfeldt P, Friberg D. Questionnaire OSA-18 has poor validity compared to polysomnography in pediatric obstructive sleep apnea. Int J Pediatr Otorhinolaryngol 2013;77(11):1864–8.
30. Lewandowski AS, Toliver-Sokol M, Palermo TM. Evidence-based review of subjective pediatric sleep measures. J Pediatr Psychol 2011;36(7):780–93.
31. Kang KT, Weng WC, Lee CH, et al. Detection of pediatric obstructive sleep apnea syndrome: history or anatomical findings? Sleep Med 2015;16(5):617–24.
32. Brietzke SE, Katz ES, Roberson DW. Can history and physical examination reliably diagnose pediatric obstructive sleep apnea/hypopnea syndrome? A systematic review of the literature. Otolaryngol Head Neck Surg 2004;131(6):827–32.
33. Feres MF, Hermann JS, Cappellette M Jr, et al. Lateral X-ray view of the skull for the diagnosis of adenoid hypertrophy: a systematic review. Int J Pediatr Otorhinolaryngol 2011;75(1):1–11.

34. Sedaghat AR, Flax-Goldenberg RB, Gayler BW, et al. A case-control comparison of lingual tonsillar size in children with and without down syndrome. Laryngoscope 2012;122(5):1165–9.

35. Caylakli F, Hizal E, Yilmaz I, et al. Correlation between adenoid-nasopharynx ratio and endoscopic examination of adenoid hypertrophy: a blind, prospective clinical study. Int J Pediatr Otorhinolaryngol 2009;73(11):1532–5.

36. Galvin JR, Rooholamini SA, Stanford W. Obstructive sleep apnea: diagnosis with ultrafast CT. Radiology 1989;171(3):775–8.

37. Boudewyns A, Verhulst S, Maris M, et al. Drug-induced sedation endoscopy in pediatric obstructive sleep apnea syndrome. Sleep Med 2014;15(12):1526–31.

38. Stuck BA, Maurer JT. Airway evaluation in obstructive sleep apnea. Sleep Med Rev 2008;12(6):411–36.

39. Revell SM, Clark WD. Late-onset laryngomalacia: a cause of pediatric obstructive sleep apnea. Int J Pediatr Otorhinolaryngol 2011;75(2):231–8.

40. Ehsan Z, Mahmoud M, Shott SR, et al. The effects of anesthesia and opioids on the upper airway: a systematic review. Laryngoscope 2016;126(1):270–84.

41. Ulualp SO, Szmuk P. Drug-induced sleep endoscopy for upper airway evaluation in children with obstructive sleep apnea. Laryngoscope 2013;123(1):292–7.

42. Shott SR, Donnelly LF. Cine magnetic resonance imaging: evaluation of persistent airway obstruction after tonsil and adenoidectomy in children with down syndrome. Laryngoscope 2004;114(10):1724–9.

43. Mahmoud M, Radhakrishman R, Gunter J, et al. Effect of increasing depth of dexmedetomidine anesthesia on upper airway morphology in children. Paediatr Anaesth 2010;20(6):506–15.

44. Ashrafian H, Toma T, Rowland SP, et al. Bariatric surgery or non-surgical weight loss for obstructive sleep apnoea? a systematic review and comparison of meta-analyses. Obes Surg 2015;25(7):1239–50.

45. Verhulst SL, Franckx H, Van Gaal L, et al. The effect of weight loss on sleep-disordered breathing in obese teenagers. Obesity 2009;17(6):1178–83.

46. Michalsky M, Reichard K, Inge T, et al. ASMBS pediatric committee best practice guidelines. Surgery for obesity and related diseases. Surg Obes Relat Dis 2012; 8(1):1–7.

47. Kalra M, Inge T, Garcia V, et al. Obstructive sleep apnea in extremely overweight adolescents undergoing bariatric surgery. Obes Res 2005;13(7):1175–9.

48. Goldbart AD, Greenberg-Dotan S, Tal A. Montelukast for children with obstructive sleep apnea: a double-blind, placebo-controlled study. Pediatrics 2012;130(3): e575–80.

49. Kheirandish-Gozal L, Bhattacharjee R, Bandla HP, et al. Antiinflammatory therapy outcomes for mild OSA in children. Chest 2014;146(1):88–95.

50. Kushida CA, Littner MR, Hirshkowitz M, et al. Practice parameters for the use of continuous and bilevel positive airway pressure devices to treat adult patients with sleep-related breathing disorders. Sleep 2006;29(3):375–80.

51. Kushida CA, Chediak A, Berry RB, et al. Clinical guidelines for the manual titration of positive airway pressure in patients with obstructive sleep apnea. J Clin Sleep Med 2008;4(2):157–71.

52. Marcus CL, Rosen G, Ward SL, et al. Adherence to and effectiveness of positive airway pressure therapy in children with obstructive sleep apnea. Pediatrics 2006;117(3):e442–51.

53. Stepanski EJ, Dull R, Basner R. CPAP titration protocols among accredited sleep disorder centers. Sleep Res 1996;25:374.

54. Fauroux B, Lavis JF, Nicot F, et al. Facial side effects during noninvasive positive pressure ventilation in children. Intensive Care Med 2005;31(7):965–9.
55. Cistulli PA, Palmisano RG, Poole MD. Treatment of obstructive sleep apnea syndrome by rapid maxillary expansion. Sleep 1998;21(8):831–5.
56. Pirelli P, Saponara M, De Rosa C, et al. Orthodontics and obstructive sleep apnea in children. Med Clin North Am 2010;94(3):517–29.
57. Holley AB, Lettieri CJ, Shah AA. Efficacy of an adjustable oral appliance and comparison with continuous positive airway pressure for the treatment of obstructive sleep apnea syndrome. Chest 2011;140(6):1511–6.
58. El-Solh AA, Moitheennazima B, Akinnusi ME, et al. Combined oral appliance and positive airway pressure therapy for obstructive sleep apnea: a pilot study. Sleep Breath 2011;15(2):203–8.
59. Pirelli P, Saponara M, Guilleminault C. Rapid maxillary expansion in children with obstructive sleep apnea syndrome. Sleep 2004;27(4):761–6.
60. Villa MP, Rizzoli A, Miano S, et al. Efficacy of rapid maxillary expansion in children with obstructive sleep apnea syndrome: 36 months of follow-up. Sleep Breath 2011;15(2):179–84.
61. Cozza P, Polimeni A, Ballanti F. A modified monobloc for the treatment of obstructive sleep apnoea in paediatric patients. Eur J Orthod 2004;26(5):523–30.
62. Villa MP, Malagola C, Pagani J, et al. Rapid maxillary expansion in children with obstructive sleep apnea syndrome: 12-month follow-up. Sleep Med 2007;8(2):128–34.
63. Huynh NT, Desplats E, Almeida FR. Orthodontics treatments for managing obstructive sleep apnea syndrome in children: a systematic review and meta-analysis. Sleep Med Rev 2016;25:84–94.
64. Baugh RF, Archer SM, Mitchell RB, et al. Clinical practice guideline: tonsillectomy in children. Otolaryngol Head Neck Surg 2011;144(1 Suppl):S1–30.
65. Marcus CL, Moore RH, Rosen CL, et al. A randomized trial of adenotonsillectomy for childhood sleep apnea. N Engl J Med 2013;368(25):2366–76.
66. Friedman M, Wilson M, Lin HC, et al. Updated systematic review of tonsillectomy and adenoidectomy for treatment of pediatric obstructive sleep apnea/hypopnea syndrome. Otolaryngol Head Neck Surg 2009;140(6):800–8.
67. Costa DJ, Mitchell R. Adenotonsillectomy for obstructive sleep apnea in obese children: a meta-analysis. Otolaryngol Head Neck Surg 2009;140(4):455–60.
68. Solares CA, Koempel JA, Hirose K, et al. Safety and efficacy of powered intracapsular tonsillectomy in children: a multi-center retrospective case series. Int J Pediatr Otorhinolaryngol 2005;69(1):21–6.
69. Brietzke SE, Gallagher D. The effectiveness of tonsillectomy and adenoidectomy in the treatment of pediatric obstructive sleep apnea/hypopnea syndrome: a meta-analysis. Otolaryngol Head Neck Surg 2006;134(6):979–84.
70. Ishii L, Roxbury C, Godoy A, et al. Does nasal surgery improve OSA in patients with nasal obstruction and OSA? A meta-analysis. Otolaryngol Head Neck Surg 2015;153(3):478.
71. Sullivan S, Li K, Guilleminault C. Nasal obstruction in children with sleep-disordered breathing. Ann Acad Med Singapore 2008;37(8):645–8.
72. Sher AE, Schechtman KB, Piccirillo JF. The efficacy of surgical modifications of the upper airway in adults with obstructive sleep apnea syndrome. Sleep 1996;19(2):156–77.
73. Friedman M, Ibrahim H, Joseph NJ. Staging of obstructive sleep apnea/hypopnea syndrome: a guide to appropriate treatment. Laryngoscope 2004;114(3):454–9.

74. Friedman M, Ibrahim HZ, Vidyasagar R, et al. Z-palatoplasty (ZPP): a technique for patients without tonsils. Otolaryngol Head Neck Surg 2004;131(1):89–100.
75. Donnelly LF, Shott SR, LaRose CR, et al. Causes of persistent obstructive sleep apnea despite previous tonsillectomy and adenoidectomy in children with down syndrome as depicted on static and dynamic cine MRI. AJR Am J Roentgenol 2004;183(1):175–81.
76. Woodson BT, Fujita S. Clinical experience with lingualplasty as part of the treatment of severe obstructive sleep apnea. Otolaryngol Head Neck Surg 1992; 107(1):40–8.
77. Clark S, Lam D, Huebi C, et al. Posterior midline glossectomy for treatment of post-adenotonsillectomy obstructive sleep apnea in children. Abstract presented at American Society of Pediatric Otolaryngology, Annual Meeting. Chicago, April 29, 2011.
78. Wootten CT, Shott SR. Evolving therapies to treat retroglossal and base-of-tongue obstruction in pediatric obstructive sleep apnea. Arch Otolaryngol Head Neck Surg 2010;136(10):983–7.
79. Prager JD, Hopkins BS, Propst EJ, et al. Oropharyngeal stenosis: a complication of multilevel, single-stage upper airway surgery in children. Arch Otolaryngol Head Neck Surg 2010;136(11):1111–5.
80. Sun GH, Harmych BM, Dickson JM, et al. Characteristics of children diagnosed as having coagulopathies following posttonsillectomy bleeding. Arch Otolaryngol Head Neck Surg 2011;137(1):65–8.
81. Roland PS, Rosenfeld RM, Brooks LJ, et al. Clinical practice guideline: polysomnography for sleep-disordered breathing prior to tonsillectomy in children. Otolaryngol Head Neck Surg 2011;145(1 Suppl):S1–15.
82. Schwengel DA, Sterni LM, Tunkel DE, et al. Perioperative management of children with obstructive sleep apnea. Anesth Analg 2009;109(1):60–75.
83. FDA Drug Safety Communication: Safety review update of codeine use in children; New boxed warning and contraindication on use after tonsillectomy and/ or adenoidectomy. 2015. Available at: http://www.fda.gov/Drugs/DrugSafety/ucm339112.htm. Accessed October 5, 2015.
84. Luna-Paredes C, Anton-Pacheco JL, Garcia Hernandez G, et al. Screening for symptoms of obstructive sleep apnea in children with severe craniofacial anomalies: assessment in a multidisciplinary unit. Int J Pediatr Otorhinolaryngol 2012; 76(12):1767–70.

# Index

*Note:* Page numbers of article titles are in **boldface** type.

Otolaryngol Clin N Am 49 (2016) 1465–1470
http://dx.doi.org/10.1016/S0030-6665(16)30183-9
0030-6665/16/$ – see front matter

oto.theclinics.com

# UNITED STATES POSTAL SERVICE®
## Statement of Ownership, Management, and Circulation
### (All Periodicals Publications Except Requester Publications)

| 1. Publication Title | 2. Publication Number | 3. Filing Date |
|---|---|---|
| OTOLARYNGOLOGIC CLINICS OF NORTH AMERICA | 466 – 550 | 9/18/2016 |

| 4. Issue Frequency | 5. Number of Issues Published Annually | 6. Annual Subscription Price |
|---|---|---|
| FEB, APR, JUN, AUG, OCT, DEC | 6 | $310.00 |

7. Complete Mailing Address of Known Office of Publication *(Not printer) (Street, city, county, state, and ZIP+4®)*
ELSEVIER INC.
360 PARK AVENUE SOUTH
NEW YORK, NY 10010-1710

Contact Person
STEPHEN R. BUSHING

Telephone *(Include area code)*
215-239-3688

8. Complete Mailing Address of Headquarters or General Business Office of Publisher *(Not printer)*
ELSEVIER INC.
360 PARK AVENUE SOUTH
NEW YORK, NY 10010-1710

9. Full Names and Complete Mailing Addresses of Publisher, Editor, and Managing Editor *(Do not leave blank)*

Publisher *(Name and complete mailing address)*
ADRIANNE BRIGIDO, ELSEVIER INC.
1600 JOHN F KENNEDY BLVD. SUITE 1800
PHILADELPHIA, PA 19103-2899

Editor *(Name and complete mailing address)*
JESSICA MCCOOL, ELSEVIER INC.
1600 JOHN F KENNEDY BLVD. SUITE 1800
PHILADELPHIA, PA 19103-2899

Managing Editor *(Name and complete mailing address)*
PATRICK MANLEY, ELSEVIER INC.
1600 JOHN F KENNEDY BLVD. SUITE 1800
PHILADELPHIA, PA 19103-2899

10. Owner *(Do not leave blank. If the publication is owned by a corporation, give the name and address of the corporation immediately followed by the names and addresses of all stockholders owning or holding 1 percent or more of the total amount of stock. If not owned by a corporation, give the names and addresses of the individual owners. If owned by a partnership or other unincorporated firm, give its name and address as well as those of each individual owner. If the publication is published by a nonprofit organization, give its name and address.)*

| Full Name | Complete Mailing Address |
|---|---|
| WHOLLY OWNED SUBSIDIARY OF REED/ELSEVIER, US HOLDINGS | 1600 JOHN F KENNEDY BLVD. SUITE 1800 PHILADELPHIA, PA 19103-2899 |

11. Known Bondholders, Mortgagees, and Other Security Holders Owning or Holding 1 Percent or More of Total Amount of Bonds, Mortgages, or Other Securities. If none, check box ▶ ☐ None

| Full Name | Complete Mailing Address |
|---|---|
| N/A | |

12. Tax Status *(For completion by nonprofit organizations authorized to mail at nonprofit rates) (Check one)*
The purpose, function, and nonprofit status of this organization and the exempt status for federal income tax purposes:
☐ Has Not Changed During Preceding 12 Months
☐ Has Changed During Preceding 12 Months *(Publisher must submit explanation of change with this statement)*

| 13. Publication Title | 14. Issue Date for Circulation Data Below |
|---|---|
| OTOLARYNGOLOGIC CLINICS OF NORTH AMERICA | JUNE 2016 |

15. Extent and Nature of Circulation

| | | | Average No. Copies Each Issue During Preceding 12 Months | No. Copies of Single Issue Published Nearest to Filing Date |
|---|---|---|---|---|
| a. Total Number of Copies *(Net press run)* | | | 610 | 638 |
| b. Paid Circulation *(By Mail and Outside the Mail)* | (1) | Mailed Outside-County Paid Subscriptions Stated on PS Form 3541 (Include paid distribution above nominal rate, advertiser's proof copies, and exchange copies) | 224 | 280 |
| | (2) | Mailed In-County Paid Subscriptions Stated on PS Form 3541 (Include paid distribution above nominal rate, advertiser's proof copies, and exchange copies) | 0 | 0 |
| | (3) | Paid Distribution Outside the Mails Including Sales Through Dealers and Carriers, Street Vendors, Counter Sales, and Other Paid Distribution Outside USPS® | 151 | 211 |
| | (4) | Paid Distribution by Other Classes of Mail Through the USPS (e.g. First-Class Mail®) | 0 | 0 |
| c. Total Paid Distribution *(Sum of 15b (1), (2), (3), and (4))* | | ▶ | 375 | 491 |
| d. Free or Nominal Rate Distribution *(By Mail and Outside the Mail)* | (1) | Free or Nominal Rate Outside-County Copies included on PS Form 3541 | 23 | 102 |
| | (2) | Free or Nominal Rate In-County Copies Included on PS Form 3541 | 0 | 0 |
| | (3) | Free or Nominal Rate Copies Mailed at Other Classes Through the USPS (e.g. First-Class Mail) | 0 | 0 |
| | (4) | Free or Nominal Rate Distribution Outside the Mail (Carriers or other means) | 0 | 0 |
| e. Total Free or Nominal Rate Distribution *(Sum of 15d (1), (2), (3) and (4))* | | ▶ | 23 | 102 |
| f. Total Distribution *(Sum of 15c and 15e)* | | ▶ | 398 | 593 |
| g. Copies not Distributed *(See Instructions to Publishers #4 (page #3))* | | ▶ | 212 | 45 |
| h. Total *(Sum of 15f and g)* | | ▶ | 610 | 638 |
| i. Percent Paid *(15c divided by 15f times 100)* | | ▶ | 94% | 83% |

* If you are claiming electronic copies, go to line 16 on page 3. If you are not claiming electronic copies, skip to line 17 on page 3.

16. Electronic Copy Circulation

| | Average No. Copies Each Issue During Preceding 12 Months | No. Copies of Single Issue Published Nearest to Filing Date |
|---|---|---|
| a. Paid Electronic Copies ▶ | 0 | 0 |
| b. Total Paid Print Copies (Line 15c) + Paid Electronic Copies (Line 16a) ▶ | 375 | 491 |
| c. Total Print Distribution (Line 15f) + Paid Electronic Copies (Line 16a) ▶ | 398 | 593 |
| d. Percent Paid (Both Print & Electronic Copies) (16b divided by 16c × 100) ▶ | 94% | 83% |

☒ I certify that 50% of all my distributed copies (electronic and print) are paid above a nominal price.

17. Publication of Statement of Ownership
☒ If the publication is a general publication, publication of this statement is required. Will be printed
in the DECEMBER 2016 issue of this publication.
☐ Publication not required.

18. Signature and Title of Editor, Publisher, Business Manager, or Owner

*Stephen R. Bushing* 

Date 9/18/2016

STEPHEN R. BUSHING - INVENTORY DISTRIBUTION CONTROL MANAGER

I certify that all information furnished on this form is true and complete. I understand that anyone who furnishes false or misleading information on this form or who omits material or information requested on the form may be subject to criminal sanctions (including fines and imprisonment) and/or civil sanctions (including civil penalties).

PS Form **3526**, July 2014 *(Page 3 of 4)* PSN 7530-01-000-9931 **PRIVACY NOTICE:** See our privacy policy on www.usps.com

PS Form **3526**, July 2014 *(Page 1 of 4 (see instructions page 4))* PSN 7530-01-000-9931 PRIVACY NOTICE: See our privacy policy on www.usps.com

PRIVACY NOTICE: See our privacy policy on www.usps.com

Printed and bound by CPI Group (UK) Ltd, Croydon, CR0 4YY

07/10/2024

01040505-0011